LONGEVITY...
SIMPLIFIED

Living A Longer, Healthier Life Shouldn't Be
Complicated

DR. HOWARD LUKS

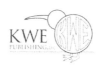

KWE
PUBLISHING

LONGEVITY...
SIMPLIFIED

Contents

Dedication

When observing the longevity space, it is clear that far too many people are going down rabbit holes and getting lost in the weeds. People are searching for magical supplements, using coffee enemas (just don't), and experimenting with potent medications that have yet to be proven to extend the human lifespan. Besides, some of the same folks who take these medications do so after sitting all day and putting down two hamburgers for lunch.

Pursuing a longer healthspan, the period of time that you are cognitively intact and physically able does not need to be complicated. I dedicate this book to those interested in your health, can look above the noise, and are looking for a reference to help achieve your goals.

Disclaimer

This book, including the text, images, and graphics, is for informational purposes only. I am not your doctor. No doctor-patient relationship is formed by reading this book. This should not be considered medical advice. No material in this book is intended to be a substitute for professional medical advice. If you have questions/concerns about some of the issues, topics, and suggestions contained herein, please discuss them with your physician. Always consult your physician with any questions after reading this book. The information in this book is to help inform your conversations with your doctor; it is not meant to replace it. Do not disregard the advice of the medical professionals treating you because of something you may have read in this book.

Foreword

I haven't told him this, but Dr Howard Luks saved my life with a simple question. Note that he didn't do it via surgery (although he's a talented surgeon), nor through personal contact (although he's eminently approachable). And he didn't do it in a TAKE MY EYE OF NEWT SUPPLEMENT THREE TIMES BEFORE LUNCH kind of way, or a IF YOU GET 30 MINUTES TOO LITTLE SLEEP YOU'LL DIE SOMETIME NEXT week health horror kind of way. It's different.

What Howard—unlike most doctors, Howard insists you call him "Howard", which turns out to be important—did was ask me a simple question: What are you optimizing for? And I didn't have a good answer to that simple question. As a runner, skier, and biker, and someone who fancied himself fit and yet was perpetually injured, I think I thought I was optimizing to run, ski, and bike.

But I wasn't. I was doing complicated fitness theater instead, a complex kind of wellness that wasn't doing me any favors, as shown by my constant injuries, mostly overuse ones from doing too much, getting hurt, taking a break, and starting all over again. That was me being stupid, and overcomplicating things.

Worse, I was tracking the wrong things. For example, I used to take great pride in how quickly I could get my heart-rate up on runs and bike rides—suffering was my mantra and metier—and I thought that's how I got fitter. And I was wrong, as I learned from discussions with Howard years ago. What I was doing was stressing my body in ways that guaranteed injuries, at best, and, at worst, could put me on the path to cardiac irregularities and even an early death. That's the path I was unknowingly on.

Howard's simple question—and this is key, the simplicity of Howard's approach—cut through all of that. By asking me what I was optimizing for—and the correct answer, in general, is healthy longevity—I was forced to reconsider what I was doing to myself, why I was doing it, and its consequences.

While the question is simple, so is his approach. Howard focuses on pulling a few physiological and metabolic levers consistently, rather than getting lost in conflicting research, expensive supplements, and pricey technological doodads. This approach is tonic in a health & wellness world full of complex, conflicting and often contradictory information, including from people who should know better.

It was the beginning of simplifying my relationship with my own health, and of focusing on a few things that matter. It was also the beginning of my personal friendship with Howard, which is one of the recent delights of my life.

But let's get back to Howard's simple question: What are you optimizing for? Ask yourself and be honest. Bringing more simplicity to what you do next could save your life.

—Dr Paul Kedrosky, Managing Partner, SK Ventures

Introduction

The average life expectancy of a healthy man is 75.1 years, and for women, it's 81 years. Sadly, for the last few years, those numbers for men have been trending lower. I suspect that if you are reading this book, you'd agree with me that it's not appealing to simply live *longer* if that means doctors' appointments each week, open-heart surgery, six medications, and being unable to get up from the floor if you fall. I think we'd both rather extend the relatively disease-free part of our lives where we can enjoy the good things and remain independent and happy for as long as possible.

As a middle-aged orthopedic surgeon and sports medicine specialist, I have spent the last few years combing through an enormous amount of data. I have done so to optimize my lifestyle strategies and prioritize my health. In recent years, I witnessed a distinct change to the subjects that have mattered most to my patients and me, from orthopedic topics like meniscus tears and osteoarthritis to living a longer, healthier, and more independent life. I have done so in order that we can all benefit from everything that I am learning along the way. Think of me as a *primary care sports doc*.

In this book, I emphasize simple, actionable strategies that work. These evidence-based strategies have been shown to improve your metabolic health, lessen the chances of suffering from many chronic diseases and early demise, and therefore increase your longevity.

These straightforward, easy strategies are:

- Create a caloric deficit, then stay lean.
- Get sleep.
- Eat real food.
- Move often, throughout the day.
- Push and pull heavy things.
- Socialize.
- Have a sense of purpose.

My goal is to improve your understanding of "simple" life-prolonging strategies that are presented in an actionable manner. Hopefully, that increases your chance of success. I am in the best shape of my life... I would love to hear you say the same thing.

The online healthcare world is loud, confusing, and sometimes wrong. Many people try to draw simple conclusions from one study when thousands of comparable studies offer different takes on enabling us to live a better life. Many people discuss approaches to improve our chances of living longer, healthier lives. We are all too easily fooled into drinking alkaline water, trying highly restrictive and unsustainable diets, or experimenting with supplements and unproven medications to improve our strength and lifespan without results or evidence of efficacy. Yes, a longer lifespan and a healthier life are attainable. We can achieve these with simple, straightforward advice backed by science.

Over the last few years, I have spent a lot of time talking about the importance of proper sleep, proper exercise, and a proper diet. And for a good reason. Let's use dementia as just one example of why this is relevant. Nearly 40 percent of dementia cases each year are preventable if we improve our diet, sleep, exercise regimen, and thus our metabolic health. And we are not talking about drastic changes that involve sweat and pain—walking even 6,000 steps per day and eating a few more nutritious foods matter. Sleeping at least seven hours a night and including bodyweight resistance exercise is quite often all the activity you need. The underlying goal for achieving a longer healthspan is *metabolic health*.

Poor metabolic health is the root cause of most chronic diseases that we suffer from. Heart disease, metabolic syndrome, stroke, dementia, type 2 diabetes, and many cancers all have poor metabolic health in common as a root cause. We will focus on this a lot throughout this book.

We are tethered to our phones. We are rushing to get the kids off to this activity or that activity. The ultra-processed foods that are omnipresent and eaten to enable our busy lifestyle contribute to the fact that we are not living longer than the generation before us for the first time in history. Many online folks get into very heated, very detailed discussions about their preferred diets, supplements, exercise patterns, and sleep patterns. Their vocal, paternalistic, and aggressive manner turns many people off. There are alternatives to the noise.

The science of longevity

The science of studying people who live to 100 years or more (centenarians) helps to show us how to live a long and healthy life. These centenarians still die of heart (cardiac) disease, etc.; they just do so 15-20 years later than everyone else. The question is: How can we do the same for ourselves?

It's one thing to live long and have a long lifespan. It's something entirely different to have a healthier lifespan--- or *healthspan*.

Your healthspan is the number of years that you live relatively disease-free—free of neurocognitive decline and free of a chronic disease burden that threatens your quality of life. Eventually, everyone will succumb to chronic disease. The goal of improving our healthspan is to keep us active, alert, and mobile to the very end.

Ultimately, we may not live longer, but we will live better. This is what we refer to as **squaring off** *your lifespan curve.* Look at the curve of lifespan versus healthspan below. For a typical lifespan curve, you hit middle age in your prime. Then you start to accumulate chronic diseases due to poor metabolic health. These diseases include hypertension, type 2 diabetes, elevated LDL, elevated triglycerides, and more. These chronic disease states start to bend our lifespan curve downward. The blue healthspan curve shows us what is achievable with improved metabolic health. We do not need to develop these chronic diseases in midlife; we can kick that can down the road 10-15 years. Thus we maintain our health, mobility, and cognition until the very end.

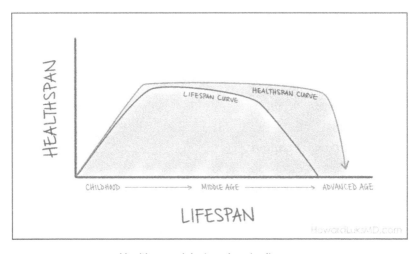

Healthspan delaying chronic disease

Our age increases horizontally from left to right. How healthy we are and feel shows up as the vertical height of the curve. As you can see, it's pretty flat in our prime years, so as we age from being very young to middle-aged, most of us enjoy reasonably good health. Then there comes the point in time where after a certain age, our health can decline. That's where the curve starts heading downward. At this point, we have a lifespan (we're still alive), but our health (and quality of life) diminishes.

My goal is to help you *square off* the lifespan curve (Weeks 2011). In the graph, that means moving the curve out along the line further to the right blue line to maintain good health for longer into our older years. If all goes to plan, we can postpone a *chronic disease burden* ten-fifteen years down the road. Centenarians follow the upper healthspan curve. In most blue zones (geographical areas with many centenarians), folks don't exercise per se. For example, they don't have a Peloton®, but instead, they are active throughout the day. They remain active, relatively disease-free, and cognitively intact well into their late nineties, and then they rapidly deteriorate or die in their sleep. That sounds far more appealing to me than an earlier onset and ongoing suffering of one or more chronic diseases. I hope this sounds more appealing to you too.

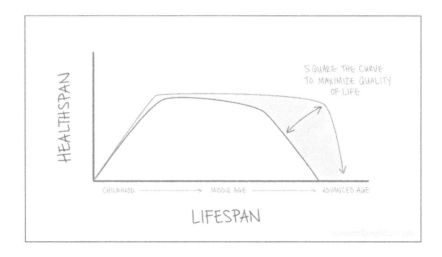

Lifespan vs. healthspan

Should extending our lives to increase our lifespan be the focus? Or should improving our healthspan and enhancing our ability to stay healthy and free of chronic disease longer be our primary goal? Our quality of life should matter more.

In my opinion, healthspan is arguably more important than lifespan. We don't want to live an extra ten years with debilitating chronic diseases. Chronic disease and frailty expose us to a widespread pathway towards our demise: falling. We see people hunched over their walker or moving along slowly with a cane. We all know people who cannot get up from a seated position independently. This is the picture of *frailty*. Frailty increases the risk of falls and increases the risk of injury following a fall. Falls are a common cause of death as we age. The fall itself might be the cause of death, or we might die due to complications of bedrest, fractures, and surgery. More than half of people with hip fractures will die within one year of the injury. Many of us don't see the effects of aging creep up on us. We think it's expected that our feet catch more on objects, stumble more often, labor to go upstairs, or be challenged to sit in a low chair as we age---it doesn't have to be.

Low-tech longevity

Let's start to explore the topic of longevity from a low-tech perspective. The longevity space can be a highly technical and challenging area to understand with any certainty. As an aging avid runner, this area interests me enormously. I'm glad to know that running may increase the chance of living longer or living better (Werner et al. 2019). But it is also essential to share the message that not everyone needs to run to be healthy.

As an orthopedic surgeon, I treat many aging athletes and

older folks who want to remain active. There has to be a tipping point where we as specialists start to step outside of our ever-present comfort zones and help you—our patients—understand the nature of human complexity with the goal of longevity and pushing off the onset of chronic disease. The healthcare system challenges providers like us and limits the desire to learn more than we were taught in medical school about subjects outside our comfort zone or specialty. I have been stepping outside that comfort zone to learn and share research on healthy aging and longevity for several years now.

I am now a 58-year-old endurance runner and amateur cyclist. I am humbled that I get to care for so many patients with salient sports injuries or arthritis. I am fascinated by the study of aging, longevity, and the concept of improving our healthspan so that I can remain active longer. This inquisitiveness enables me to focus on holding off the onset of chronic disease for 10-15 years longer than our current lifespan curve predicts. I'm not selfish in my efforts. I want to share this information with you in a way that I hope is easy to understand and incorporate into your plan to live better.

How do we increase our healthspan?

So, the question is: How do we increase our healthspan well into our eighties and beyond? Anti-aging and longevity research has been quite the rage for a while now. There are thousands of studies with varying takes on what might enable us to live a better life. The scientific literature on longevity is fascinating. It is also very confusing. Hopefully, after reading this book, you will under-stand that no single action, medication, diet, or supplement will extend your life.

As mentioned earlier, the achievable goal to lengthen your healthspan is improving your metabolic health. You are *metaboli-cally healthy* when you have ideal blood sugar levels, insulin levels, blood pressure, blood lipids (triglycerides, high-density lipoprotein (HDL), cholesterol), and no abdominal obesity. There are plenty of "normal" weight individuals who are not metabolically healthy. In addition, there are plenty of people who are overweight but are metabolically healthy. You do not need to be thin to be in good metabolic health.

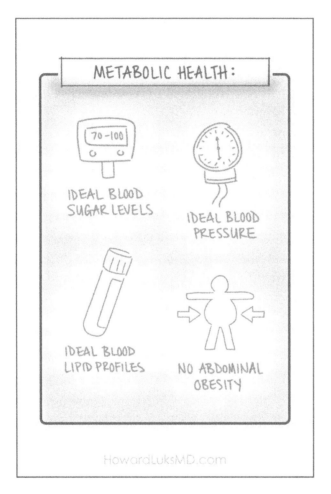

Many centenarians have a genetic advantage. They may have "won" the genetic lottery and have the genes and a genetic phenotype that protects their health well into their eighties and nineties. But we can achieve similar outcomes (maybe not living to 100— but closer) by being *metabolically fit*. Being metabolically fit lowers your risk for developing heart (cardiac) disease, cognitive decline (dementia), stroke, type 2 diabetes, and cancer. These chronic diseases all have a basis or foundation in poor metabolic health. Certain habits like smoking, stress, poor dietary habits, lack of sleep, and exercise also contribute.

There are many reports of people reversing insulin resistance, heart disease, and fatty liver with changes to their diet and proper exercise. Whether you're in your thirties, fifties, or beyond, it is never too late to address your metabolic health.

Some of the significant factors critical to maintaining a long healthspan are a combination of lifestyle, sleep, diet, and movement and avoiding toxic habits like smoking. Many non-physical factors are also important, such as stress management, optimism, laughing, being socially connected, and feeling a sense of purpose and community.

I have been an orthopedic surgeon for nearly 25 years. I have returned many athletes to the playing field with my knife and replaced more knees than I can count throughout my career. Despite that, I am now delighted to help entire families improve their health with lifestyle, exercise, and dietary modifications. Those are, by far, some of the biggest success stories in my practice. Returning people to a path of being metabolically healthy will impact their entire life and the lives of those they bring along on their journey. We will go into detail on metabolic health in chapter 2.

Contrary to popular belief among some of my peers, people will often engage if they understand *why* they should do something and *how* to accomplish it. Over the last decade, I have chosen to optimize my overall health and the overall health of those I treat. What often becomes evident in interactions with my patients is that most of them want to change their diets (within reason) and want to exercise more. They are delighted to learn that they can continue to eat many of the foods they enjoy. They are especially pleased to know that exercise does not need to be sweaty and painful. No one wants to continue their march down a path towards heart disease, stroke, disability, or neurocognitive decline. Information is empowering. Knowing why we need to change and how our actions can affect that change is powerful and often motivating.

Metabolic health matters—even if you don't lose weight. This book was created to help you optimize your metabolic health. I will take you through many lifestyles, sleep, diet, movement, and exercise factors that can make meaningful improvements to your healthspan.

The journey has to start somewhere. What will spark your lightbulb moment? Make today the first day on your journey towards metabolic health and longevity.

You in? Then, let's get on with this.

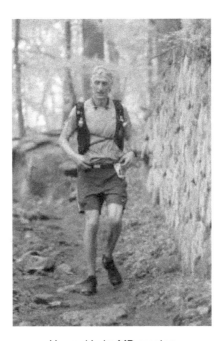

Howard Luks MD running

Chapter 1
LONGEVITY GOALS AND WHY THEY'RE ESSENTIAL, WHATEVER YOUR AGE

Your reasons for wanting to live a longer, healthier life may be to ward off dementia, type 2 diabetes, heart disease, or other chronic diseases. Or maybe it's to stay independent and robust as long as possible. Whatever your reason, this book will show you how likely it is to positively impact and lengthen your healthspan. Many straightforward, actionable strategies help, including:

- Creating a caloric deficit, then staying lean.
- Getting sleep.
- Eating real food.
- Moving often, throughout the day.
- Pushing and pulling heavy things.
- Socializing.
- Having a sense of purpose.

Before we go into all of these lifestyle factors under our control, let's first talk about another physical benefit linked to improved metabolic health and a longer healthspan: our waistlines.

Another benefit of an improved healthspan

Beyond health, some of the added bonuses of living a longevity-focused lifestyle are physical benefits. For example, we may be well aware of the "beer" or "menopause" belly. Abdominal fat can be part of the *metabolic syndrome* (or metabolic dysfunction), which we're going to discuss in a lot more detail in chapter 2. Metabolic syndrome includes insulin resistance, high blood pressure (hypertension), high triglycerides, and abdominal obesity. Abdominal fat is toxic because people with belly fat usually also have insulin resistance, systemic inflammation, and high blood pressure. Abdominal fat is metabolically different than the fat under your skin. Your metabolic health matters. Your metabolism affects every system in your body, including your muscles, tendons, and joints.

All of our bodies' processes are connected; this is why you need to know that metabolic syndrome is not four distinct diseases. Treating just one of them (insulin resistance *or* hypertension *or* high triglycerides *or* abdominal obesity) won't make it get better. Medications might control these diseases, but they do not cure them.

The best way to get rid of a "beer" or "menopause" belly is to improve your metabolic fitness. This means following the recommendations in this book to sleep better, eat better, and move more. Together these will enhance your metabolic fitness and all of its effects on health and longevity—whether you can physically see them or not.

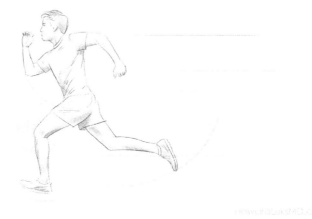

How DNA is linked to healthspan (telomeres and epigenetics)

Your DNA (the genes in each of our cells) is linked to your healthspan in several ways. One is the genetic code you were given from your parents. Next comes the subject of epigenetics. All of your DNA isn't actively utilized at the same time. Only a small portion is. Your diet, health, exercise patterns will affect which genes in your DNA are turned on and which are turned off. Another aspect of our DNA that might affect our health is how long our telomeres are. Longer telomeres *might be* associated with a longer healthspan and less of a lifelong burden due to chronic disease.

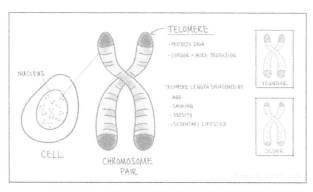

A *telomere* is a protective cap on the end of a strand of your DNA. The longer the protective cap, the safer your DNA is from being damaged. Telomeres shorten as we age. They also shorten if we smoke, if we are obese, or if we are sedentary. Your telomere length might give us a clue about your *biological* age (Benetos et al. 2001). This means that someone who is seventy years old but has longer telomeres than other people their age is *biologically* younger than their peers. Telomere length is diminished in people with chronic disease. Your telomere length might also be predictive of your risk of having cardiac disease. Scientists now believe that healthy long telomeres might promote healthier aging by keeping us healthy for a more extended period. Scientists have been trying to find ways to increase the length of these protective caps for a while now.

Genetics also plays an inevitable role in our healthspan. Both from a Mendelian perspective (the genetic cards you were dealt) and from an epigenetic perspective. Epigenetics is quite fascinating. *Epigenetics* is how the DNA code you were born with is *expressed* in you. So, you may have a perfectly normal strand of DNA, but due to telomere length or some other damage, the protein or enzyme that your DNA codes for is altered. This can lead to degradation of your cellular function and aging. As mentioned, telomeres are protective caps on your DNA, and the longer they are, the lower your biological age. The length of your telomeres can be affected by several things. On average, the longer people have exercised, the longer their telomeres appear to be. This is not a binary issue, though, and other factors beyond exercise come into play. Our telomere length may not be as long as we would want it to be because of genetics, lifestyle, dietary issues, and other toxic habits. There are many things you can do to increase your healthspan, beginning with sleep.

Sleep for longevity

Below is an exhaustive list of systems in your body that are not negatively affected by a lack of sleep:

1. ...

Sleep is crucial for our overall health and well-being. It has been a genetically well-conserved process across all living beings from the beginning of time. Poor sleep can lead to heart disease, cognitive decline, dementia, insulin resistance, and a decrease in your immunity.

As I said, there are no biological processes in our bodies that aren't negatively affected by a loss of sleep. We will go more in-depth about the importance of sleep and steps to improve it in chapter 5.

Eating for longevity

A typical Western lifestyle and diet are not likely to help you achieve your healthspan goals. You cannot outrun, out-exercise, or medicate away a poor diet. Your lifestyle choices and decisions around your sleep, diet, exercise, and more lay out the appropriate foundation on which you can build your healthy longevity program.

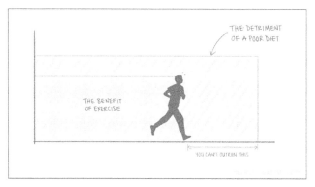

Fad diets are the rage but typically do not lead to sustained lifestyle changes. Eating real food, less of it, and getting enough fiber in your diet to support your gut are advantageous. Despite the banter in certain social circles, monitoring your LDL, triglycerides, cholesterol, HbA1c, homocysteine, uric acid, and other basic biomarkers (substances in your blood that we can monitor) is essential. Over time, this monitoring gives you a snapshot of how your dietary, sleep, and exercise habits shape your risk of developing chronic disease. We will go over these medical tests when we talk about determining your metabolic health in chapter 2.

The earlier you focus on your diet and other contributors to longevity in life, the more likely you are to live a longer, disease-free, independent life. Chapter 6 will share tips and recommendations for a nutritious way to become more metabolically healthy.

Staying active for longevity

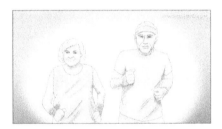

I always hear from folks who think they need to run hard or ride their Peloton® hard to achieve fitness. I also hear from many who think they need to sweat on a treadmill to derive metabolic health benefits. This approach is not necessary. If the thoughts of sweat and pain turn you off, this book is for you. On the other hand, if you do enjoy those workouts, this book is also for you! Throughout the book, we will talk about realistic expectations for physical movement to increase your metabolic fitness and longevity and why it becomes more and more important to keep moving as we age.

For me, trail running has long been my happy place. Any form of running enables me to start my day invigorated and ready to go. Regular exercise is associated with many upsides. Exercising so that we can live longer is likely a draw for you.

Simply put, the best exercise is the one that you will enjoy and continue pursuing because you enjoy it. Different exercises offer different benefits, although you will derive aerobic benefit any time your heart rate rises.

If your goal is to achieve metabolic health, exercise does not need to be painful and sweaty.

Walking

Research shows that we only need to walk for 15-20 minutes a day to see the benefits of exercise. For many of us, short walks throughout the day might be enough. For others, it will not be. Research shows that a single bout of exercise followed by a day on the couch doesn't improve markers of metabolic health. It's better to be active all day. For example, you can go for a walk in the morning, park in the farthest parking spot or take the stairs when you go out, then have another walk after dinner. Move more, move often, occasionally with ferocious intent. Moving more often throughout the day is healthier than one bout of exercise in the morning, followed by a completely sedentary day on the couch or at a desk.

Swimming

You may love to swim. Swimming provides an excellent combined aerobic and resistance-based exercise. You will maintain muscle mass, improve your heart function, lower your blood pressure, lower your cholesterol, and improve your blood sugar (glucose) management with any aerobic exercise program.

Cycling and running

Cycling and running are great exercise programs. They offer the same benefits as other aerobic activities, but you will still benefit from adding in resistance exercises.

Mary was a 76-year-old woman I met at the starting line of a race a few years ago. She's been running for decades. She loved to run for many different reasons, but she found it increasingly more challenging to finish a course in the allotted time. She had no intention of stopping and was very interested in meeting in my office one day to address strategies to help her maintain her running habits deep into her elder years.

Over the last two decades of treating athletes of all ages, it has become apparent that older athletes are just as driven as younger superstars. They thrive on the thrill of a race, regardless of pace. They thrive on the way it makes them feel, and they will go to any length to protect their time on the road or the trail.

The earlier in life that you focus on physical activity, whether your goal is to be an athlete or not, the more likely you are to lengthen your healthspan. Chapter 4 looks at aerobic exercise, chapter 7 focuses on the benefits of resistance exercise, and chapter 8 focuses on how to progress your fitness goals.

Muscle strength for longevity

A complete exercise program has four pillars: aerobic training, resistance training, balance training, and high-intensity training (HIT). These work together to improve your metabolic health and diminish your risks for insulin resistance, type 2 diabetes, heart (cardiovascular) disease, stroke, high blood pressure (hypertension), high blood lipids, age-related muscle loss (sarcopenia), etc.

During our more formative years, we laced up and ran outside. We didn't worry about balance, strength, muscle tone, and energy. As we age, these become salient issues to address proactively.

Reducing injuries by improving balance

Your mobility and strength are tightly linked to your healthspan. This means, for example, that you should be able to squat down and pick something up without assistance. This is a marker for resiliency and the ability to survive and recover from a fall. Being able to squat, crouch down, and reach the ground has been linked to longer, better healthspans (Yeh et al. 2018).

As we age, our ability to balance and stabilize ourselves diminishes. This is a far more serious problem than most people realize. While chronic disease sets us up for a diminished healthspan, injuries sustained due to a fall and the downtime to recover from those injuries significantly affect our health and longevity. Falls can lead to frailty and the end of independent living.

Diminishing our fall risk starts with an active balance training program. These do not need to be elaborate gym-based programs, as there are plenty of balance exercises we can perform in the comfort of our home. Standing on one leg for 30 seconds can be challenging enough (if so, be sure to have something to hold on to as you build your balance). When that becomes easy, perturb the system by moving your arms around while one leg is off the ground. You will notice an improvement in your balance and control within a few weeks. Switch legs every minute. Carry small cans or 1-pound weights in your hands when bodyweight alone becomes too easy.

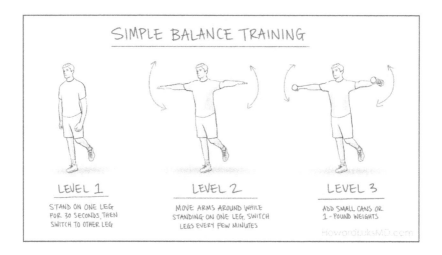

You will feel more surefooted and confident after these exercises. Your risk of falling will diminish with this program, and you will have further reduced the risk of injury after a fall with your resistance exercise program.

Recovering from exercise and injuries

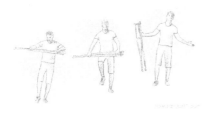

Consequences of inactivity or rest on our health

"You should rest." How many times have you heard that? From an orthopedic perspective, the term *rest* is a relative term. If you are used to running 30 miles per week, and something bothers you, *rest* might mean running 10-15 miles per week. If you're used to running 10-minute miles, then you may need to run 12-minute miles. The same goes for resistance training. Absolute rest and ceasing all activities are seldom necessary. You will rapidly lose the aerobic or strength benefits of your training. A few weeks of no exercise, and you are set back months in terms of the level at which you were training. The consequences of even a few weeks of inactivity or rest are dramatic. Your body's chemistry changes, your muscles change, and your heart and lungs decondition significantly.

The concept of *recovery* is poorly understood among average runners and cyclists alike. Have you noticed that the day after a particularly long walk, ride or jog, your heart rate is a little higher, or perhaps you're a little short of breath? Your body is telling you that it needs to have a lighter day. Recovery, just like rest, is a relative term. If you rode your bike 40 miles the day before, a recovery ride might only be 4 miles. If you jogged 5 miles, then a recovery day might be a 1-mile walk. At least one or two days a week, you should let your body completely rest from resistance or pushing your aerobic thresholds. That doesn't mean you can't hike or take a walk. It simply means that you need to let your heart and muscles recover and repair themselves from your activity over the past week.

Rest and recovery are different. Rest is a relative term. Respect your body's need to recover.

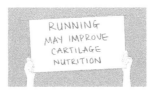

Running improves the health of cartilage

Exercise does not cause osteoarthritis

Many people are concerned that exercise can increase their risk for osteoarthritis. In fact, it is quite the opposite. Runners have a lower incidence of osteoarthritis when compared to a matched group of less active peers. It turns out that your cartilage (the cushioning) in your knees thrives on the cyclical loading of running. If you already have osteoarthritis or some degeneration in your knee, then let pain be your guide. It may be best to cross-train with swimming or cycling if your arthritis is advanced enough that running simply hurts too much to pursue.

Yes, you can exercise if you have knee osteoarthritis. Exercise and strength training might delay the need for you to think about knee replacement surgery. Weakness in our legs might predispose us to the development of osteoarthritis. Exercise can minimize the risk of developing osteoarthritis because arthritis development is not a *mechanical* process.

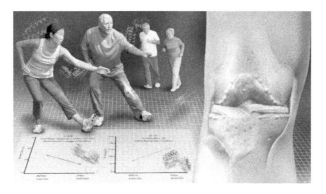

Exercising with knee osteoarthritis is OK

Osteoarthritis development is a complex *biological* process. The cartilage or cushioning in your knee is not worn away by moving it. That grinding sound is rarely a sign of something serious going on. More often than not, the grinding and clicking are due to inflammation. Once again, osteoarthritis is a biological process. There are many chemicals, cytokines, and proteins in our joints. Some of those chemicals might be harmful to our cartilage. Exercise, and even running, can decrease the concentration of the nasty chemicals in our knees that lead to cartilage damage.

Is it OK to exercise with pain?

As we age, this is a fundamental issue to understand. Many of us have discomfort with certain activities. Most of us are stiff and have discomfort when we wake up in the morning. More often than not, you do not need to stop exercising if you were told you have osteoarthritis, especially if you don't experience moderate-to-severe pain. Keep reading to see how to use pain as your guide. Plainly stated, there are virtually no overuse tendon issues treated with absolute rest. Our tendons can start to bother us for many reasons. In general, our tendons hate surprise parties and vacations. They respond poorly to abrupt changes in activity levels. But stopping an exercise program is rarely in your best interest. Stopping your exercises will result in loss of heart health, loss of muscle mass, loss of endurance and make it harder to get back into your exercise regimen.

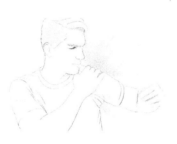

Aches and pains are commonplace and are often just a mild annoyance or nuisance. Exercise or physiotherapy is often the best way to address them. Again, absolute rest is rarely the correct answer. Now that comes with a caveat. Think of a pain scale from 0-10, with 0 being no pain; if you have pain during activity and rate it under 4, it is generally OK to continue exercising. By all means, if you have pain that concerns you, then you should stop and see your practitioner.

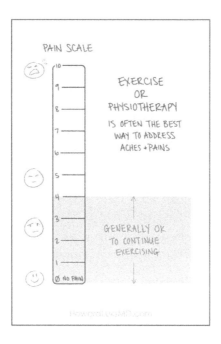

If you do choose to see a doctor, you must remember to ask if rest is necessary. If they say yes, ask for how long and the potential downsides of *not* resting. For example, groin pain with specific exercises like running could potentially indicate a stress fracture of the hip. You should not exercise with a stress fracture of your hip. But groin pain can also be due to a muscle strain. The proper treatment for a muscle strain could be to stretch and strengthen it. So do not be afraid to ask your doctor pointed questions about what they believe the source of your pain is, how they will prove it, and whether or not continuing to exercise puts you at risk of developing a more severe injury. If you have pain, physical therapy is often effective at treating the pain associated with tendon issues and degenerative tears in your knee, shoulder, hip, and elbow.

In the end, the vast majority of patients I see do not need to stop exercising and should not stop their exercises for mild aches and pains. You want to avoid potentially problematic issues like a stress fracture, but you never want the risk of the treatment to be higher than the risk of the injury. So take it upon yourself to ask what your doctor believes might be the cause of your pain. Have them clarify if any further tests are needed. Ask them if rest is absolutely necessary. You will need a solid plan and goal if you aim to continue your exercise pursuits for years to come.

Overall, it's clear that sleep, eating right, and exercising are critical to achieving your best possible health. Regarding the types of exercise we should pursue, we will cover practices to improve metabolic health and reduce age-related muscle loss (sarcopenia). Improving our aerobic capacity, metabolic health, and strength will require both aerobic and resistance exercises. Balance training becomes an essential component of your overall exercise program because it minimizes your risk of falling. Before you start an exercise program, speak with your doctor.

Take-Home Points:

1. Improving your healthspan and longevity are important goals regardless of your age.
2. Metabolic health matters. It is the root cause of most major diseases.
3. You do not need to be at your ideal body weight to achieve metabolic fitness.
4. One bout of exercise will drop your blood pressure for up to 24 hours.
5. Getting enough sleep is critical.
6. Exercise comes in many forms; walking and other low-impact forms of exercise can improve a person's fitness and health.
7. Movement matters. Move often throughout the day.
8. Exercising when you have osteoarthritis is ok.

Chapter 2
METABOLIC HEALTH IS YOUR KEY TO A LONGER HEALTHSPAN

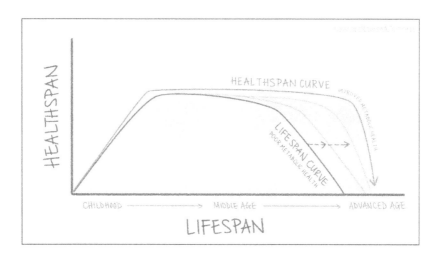

It turns out that only 12 percent of Americans are considered "metabolically healthy" (Araújo et al. 2019). You are metabolically healthy when you have ideal insulin levels, blood sugar, blood pressure, and blood lipids like triglycerides, high-density lipoprotein (HDL), and cholesterol.

For a longer healthspan, we need to focus on metabolic *health* instead of focusing on managing metabolic *disease*.

Metabolic health is an *area under the curve* issue. An *area under the curve* issue means that time is a crucial variable. For example, having a high LDL (low-density lipoprotein) level for 20 years is worse than two years. That's because your blood vessels have been exposed to those LDL particles for more time (thus having more area under the curve). Being exposed to these abnormal metabolic markers for years increases your risk of developing chronic diseases like heart disease. Unlike with the healthspan curve, having more area under the curve due to elevated lipids, insulin, blood glucose, etc., means that the longer you are metabolically unhealthy, the worse the consequences. In other words, don't try to convince yourself that you have another decade or two to focus on this.

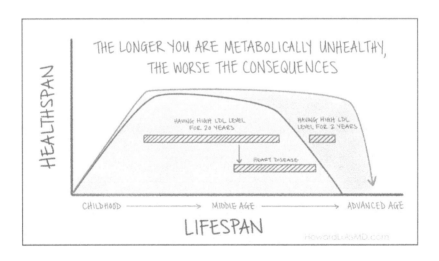

Being metabolically healthy is not about speeding up a "slow" metabolism. You can't do that because your hypothalamus is in control. Your hypothalamus is a tiny area in your brain that regulates many processes like hunger. Your body tends to keep your basal metabolic rate (the energy you expend at rest) reasonably stable. It doesn't matter whether you are a hunter-gatherer or a sedentary American. Our basal metabolic rates are remarkably similar. Your metabolism is cruel that way. You can improve your metabolic health by improving your diet, increasing your muscle mass, moving more, moving often, and increasing your aerobic fitness, all of which we'll discuss in detail later on.

My interests in metabolism were shaped by the recent research showing just how important being in good metabolic health is. This is why we always say that you can't outrun, out-exercise, or medicate away a poor diet. Our body's processes are connected in ways we are only starting to understand. Exercise is great but not as good for us as it could be if we also focus on other issues that affect our metabolic health.

Let me reiterate: You can't outrun your fork!

Metabolic health helps your joints, too. From an orthopedic surgery and sports medicine perspective, poor metabolic health and metabolic disease have been proven to affect knee pain, our rotator cuff and even increase our risk of developing osteoarthritis. Really? Yes! Too many people—even some orthopedic surgeons—think that our joints wear out from mechanical wear or cumulative force when it comes to osteoarthritis. Granted, that does play a minimal role, as does injury, but given the epidemic of fatty liver disease and other metabolic diseases such as type 2 diabetes, our metabolic health may play a much more significant role than we think (Courties et al. 2017).

The more we learn about various disease processes and their effects on us as a whole, the more critical it becomes to manage our metabolic health actively. It's time that we emphasize the importance of forks over knives—and forks over pills. As you age, your knees, shoulders, low back, and hips will thank you for maintaining metabolic health.

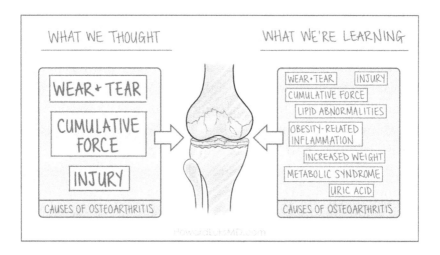

YOUR METABOLIC HEALTH will also affect how much joint pain you experience once osteoarthritis has started. People with lipid (LDL, HDL, triglyceride) abnormalities are at higher risk for tendon injuries, too. Scientific studies have shown an association between rotator cuff tears and an abnormal lipid profile (Lai and Gagnier 2018). Other research has found high cholesterol in people with rotator cuff tears (Abboud and Kim 2010).

I hope you start seeing the connection between your metabolic health and orthopedic or sports medicine wellness. Granted, correcting your lipid profile isn't going to reverse your arthritis, but it just might delay the onset of your next joint problem—and extend your healthspan.

Beyond your blood lipids, inflammation is another related troublemaker that is a pillar of metabolic syndrome. *Systemic* inflammation (inflammation throughout your body) can affect how you perceive pain—for example, people with diabetes experience more pain with orthopedic issues than people without diabetes. People with elevated blood (serum) markers for inflammation have a higher chance of having pain due to osteoarthritis (Ioan-Facsinay and Kloppenburg 2018).

So, elevated cholesterol and LDL increase your risk for inflammation, and that will increase your pain. Some people live very productive lives with osteoarthritis and have very little pain. Other people have mild arthritis, yet they have severe pain. Perhaps our metabolic profile has a role in this. It certainly appears that it does.

Am I metabolically healthy?

Far too often, we use outward appearance or weight to view if someone appears healthy. That method doesn't work. "Normal weight obesity" is a real threat to some who have a normal weight but poor muscle mass and poor metabolic health. This is why you must know your blood test values too. Metabolic health is much more than just our weight.

The biomarkers listed below are ones that we should check annually to help determine your metabolic health. Talk with your doctor about these tests:

- Waist Circumference: <102 cm for men or 88 cm for women/<40 inches for men or 35 inches for women.
- Systolic Blood Pressure: <120 mmHg (when it comes to your blood pressure readings, systolic matters the most).
- Diastolic Blood Pressure: <80 mmHg.
- Fasting Glucose: <100 mg/dL.
- HbA1c: <5.7%.
- Triglycerides: <150 mg/dL.
- HDL-C: >=40/50 mg/dL men/women.
- Cholesterol preferably under 180.
- Lp(a): Responsible for perhaps 15% of heart attacks at a young age. Normal levels are under 30 mg/dl.
- ApoB vs. LDLc: ApoB tracks your risk of heart disease better than LDL- levels under 70 are optimal.
- Uric acid: Uric acid levels can indicate high blood

pressure and issues other than only gout. Levels under 5 are optimal.

- Homocysteine: Some studies speak to the risk of dementia and arterial damage if these levels are high. In a healthy person, homocysteine levels are around five to 15 micromoles per liter (mcmol/L).
- Resting pulse: In general, the lower your resting heart rate, the healthier you are.

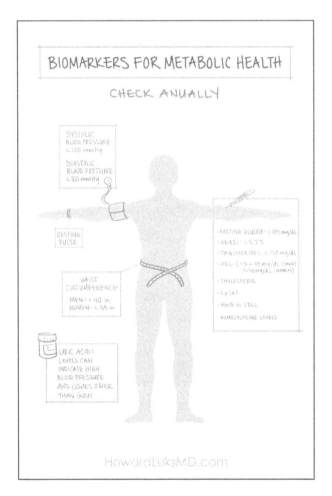

Make sure you know your biomarkers. If something is off, ask what you can do to correct it. For example, your cardiologist might recommend vitamin B or folate supplements if you have high homocysteine. Or, if you need to drop your cholesterol levels, you may need to increase your fiber intake. It's true! A high fiber intake can lower your cholesterol level significantly.

Data and scientific papers are starting to reveal that almost all chronic diseases share a common cause: metabolic dysfunction. A common cause of metabolic dysfunction is our diet, and more accurately, the number of calories we consume and the foods which contribute to that caloric burden.

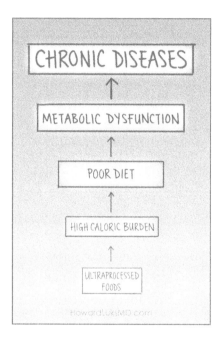

What is metabolic syndrome (metabolic dysfunction)?

As previously mentioned, *metabolic syndrome* is the combination of insulin resistance, hypertension, high triglycerides, and abdominal obesity. A pet peeve is that most people are told they have one or more of these and go home from their doctor's appointments thinking they have four different diseases. If this is you, you do not have four various conditions. You have one. In reality, you have metabolic syndrome, which is the downstream effect of a lack of metabolic fitness. Most of the issues that surface due to poor metabolic health also lead to problems that dramatically affect our longevity, like type 2 diabetes and heart disease. Therefore, this book was written to help you focus on and achieve metabolic health. Achieving metabolic health will help you address your type 2 diabetes risk, hypertension, heart disease risk, stroke risk, and so on.

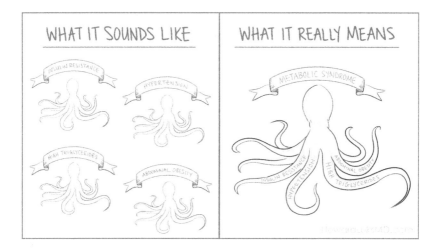

One of the root causes of poor metabolic health is poorly functioning mitochondria (which we'll talk about in chapter 8). Improve the health of your mitochondria with a few "simple" tips, and you start to improve your metabolic health, and thus your longevity. In this book, we will tie this all together. By correcting the metabolic health issues, you could potentially reverse the metabolic syndrome.

How to improve your metabolic health

The lower your waistline, pulse, blood pressure, triglycerides, and glucose, the better chance you can prolong the time before the onset of chronic disease. In other words, by improving your metabolic health, you are extending your healthspan.

The forces seem like they are stacked against us. Drug companies do not benefit if you achieve metabolic fitness on your own without their pills. Big food is not our friend.

Evolutionarily speaking, we were not meant to have food available 24 hours a day, 7 days a week, 365 days a year, especially when that food is filled with substances that contribute to metabolic disease. Ultra-processed foods lead to more significant gains in fat than natural foods with the same number of calories. We go into detail about healthy food choices in chapter 6.

There is no magic diet. There is no magical supplement. You will not burn more fat from eating a pill you purchased online. Your gut is your second brain. We need to take care of it. Our intestine synthesizes two essential neurotransmitters—serotonin and dopamine—which your brain uses to communicate between nerve cells. Proper gut health is of paramount importance when it comes to maintaining true metabolic health. Bacteria in your gut produce short-chain fatty acids from breaking down fiber. Those short-chain fatty acids repair many tissues in our bodies, decrease our risk of colon cancer, decrease inflammation, improve our cardiac risk profile, and might decrease our dementia risk. We will explore gut health later on in more detail.

Step 1. Calculate your basal metabolic rate (BMR)

One goal when pursuing metabolic health is to try to be at a "normal" weight. But as I mentioned earlier, you can be overweight and still possess proper metabolic health.

If weight loss is on your bucket list, the only way to achieve weight loss is by acquiring a caloric deficit. A caloric deficit is when you take in fewer calories than you burn each day. The number of calories you burn each day is your basal metabolic rate (BMR).

It doesn't matter which diet you consider using to reach this goal. Weight loss can be achieved with low-fat diets, high-fat diets, high-carb diets, and low-carb diets. As we will discuss later, the key is to eat real food and leave the ultra-processed foods in the store. Then we need to try to achieve a caloric deficit. You can only achieve weight loss from a caloric deficit, so choose a diet that works for you. Track your calories, and try to eat fewer calories than you burn each day.

Find the diet that works for you. It may not be the same diet that worked for your friend. Whichever foods you choose to form a diet plan, keep in mind that you must find the foods palatable and enjoyable. Otherwise, your new dietary strategy will not work.

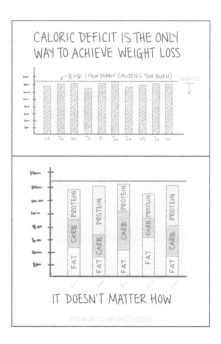

Figuring out how many calories you burn isn't challenging. When you know how many calories you burn for your basal metabolic rate (the energy we expend at rest) and how many more calories you burn for your activities, you know the maximum number of calories you need every day. Once you know your calorie needs every day, you can achieve a caloric deficit by consuming slightly less than that or becoming more active. Starvation will not work in the long run. Starvation triggers potent pathways in our brains that will eventually cause us to eat more.

Most men have a BMR of 1,600 to 1,800 kCals a day. Most women have a BMR of 1,550 kCals a day. Remember, this represents the calories you need to perform essential bodily functions. You need to add the calories your burned from activities to know the total number of calories you burned.

For a more precise calculation of your total daily caloric burn, you can use the following formulas:

For males, use the following equation to calculate your basal metabolic rate (BMR):

- 66 + (6.2 x weight in pounds) + (12.7 x height in inches) – (6.76 x age) = Basal metabolic rate for males.

For example, a 40-year-old, 180 pound, 6-foot-tall man has a basal metabolic rate of 1,826. This means that, at rest, they'll burn approximately 1,826 calories in a day (equation: 66 + (6.2 x 180) + (12.7 x 72) – (6.76 x 40) = 1,826).

For females, use the following equation:

- 65.1 + (4.35 x weight in pounds) + (4.7 x height in inches) – (4.7 x age) = Basal metabolic rate for females.

For example, a 40-year-old, 150-pound, 5 foot 6-inch-tall woman has a basal metabolic rate of 1,429.8 (equation: 65.1 + (4.35 x 150) + (4.7 x 66) – (4.7×40) = 1,429.8).

Step 2. Factor in the additional calories you burn.

From there, you must figure out your activity level to understand how many additional calories you need over and above merely functioning at rest (BMR). The activity level factors are as follows:

- 1.2 if you are sedentary (little to no exercise).
- 1.375 if you are lightly active (light exercise 1–3 days per week).
- 1.55 if you are moderately active (moderate exercise 3–5 days per week).
- 1.725 if you are very active (challenging exercise 6–7 days per week).
- 1.9 if you are extra active (very hard exercise, training, or work a physical job).

For example, someone who walks all day for their job would have an activity level of 1.725.

An office worker who walks several times a week for exercise would have an activity level of 1.55.

Step 3. Determine how many calories you need every day—at the most—to maintain your current weight

Putting everything together:

- BMR x activity level = the calories you need to maintain your current weight.

The example of the 180-pound male who's moderately active will need 2,830 calories to maintain their weight (equation: 1826 (BMR) x 1.55 (activity level) = 2,830 calories).

The example of the 150-pound female who's extra active will need 2,717 calories to maintain their weight (equation: 1,429.8 (BMR) x 1.9 (activity level) = 2,717 calories).

Step 4: Now you know how to create a caloric deficit.

Your everyday diet has areas where small wins are achievable. The cream in your coffee, the snacking before bedtime, the donut with your coffee in the morning all count. These little 100-200 calorie wins add up dramatically over time.

I don't want to recommend a specific diet because your genetics and gut microbiome (bacteria) may respond differently to various diets. Choosing the proper diet and foods is an individual choice. You have options. Different diets work for different people. The diet that works best for us is the one that we can sustain. Diets rich in natural foods, including vegetables, fruit, lean meat, complex carbs, and grains, appear best. Elimination diets, in the long run, are often unsuccessful and may be unhealthy. The Mediterranean diet is a good example of a diet backed by a wealth of scientific studies.

Will "keto" work for you? I don't know. And the online talking heads don't know either. Will a low-carb diet work best for you? Maybe. A low-carb diet might be perfect, especially if you have diabetes or a fatty liver. If you have diabetes, you need to approach these diets with the help of your doctor.

Is the Paleo or meat-only diet safe? I don't know the answer to that, either. Twenty years of data show that exposure to animal fat may not be very healthy for us over the long term. I will not listen to any paternalistic online guru or talking head because they simply do not have the data to know which diet is best. Sadly those high-quality studies haven't been done. I'm also not willing to dismiss the saturated fat/LDL/cardiac disease hypothesis, which has a lot of data supporting it.

Be careful what you read. As you will see in chapter 6, I recommend that you stick with real food, cook and prepare your meals, and leave the food industry's junk in the supermarket. Toss the crap in your kitchen, walk outside, let's eat real food. Head to your kitchen with an oversized garbage bag or two.

Sarcopenia should be a four-letter word.

If you are asked to describe an older person, what sort of

words come to mind? For many, the answer probably includes something along the lines of *frail* or *weak*. And it turns out there's a reason for this: sarcopenia. *Sarcopenia* is a fancy word for the natural process of age-related loss of lean muscle mass.

Starting in our thirties, we naturally lose a percentage of our muscle mass every year. At around fifty years of age, you lose about one percent of your muscle mass per year. By the time you are in your seventies and eighties, the loss of muscle mass can be profound.

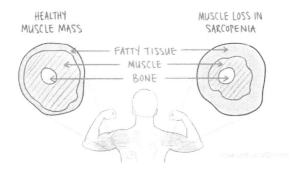

Sarcopenia: age-related muscle loss

If you're a health and fitness enthusiast like myself, then this information may seem quite depressing. Luckily, sarcopenia is not inevitable. Sarcopenia is avoidable and treatable.

The causes of sarcopenia are debated, but it appears to be multifactorial, with many related factors contributing to the decline. For example, "decreased physical activity, lower hormone excretion, nutritional deficits, and possibly chronic inflammation" contribute (Siparsky et al., 2014). One primary reason for sarcopenia is that our body cannot synthesize new muscle protein as we did when we were younger. In other words, we have a reduced capacity to manufacture new *muscle proteins*. Combine this loss of new muscle protein with increased resistance to insulin (the hormone that lowers blood sugar), systemic inflammation due to chronic disease, and a decreased basal metabolic rate; the result is less lean muscle mass.

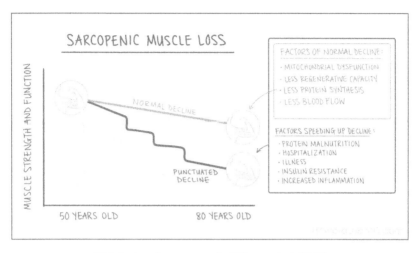

Risk factors for sarcopenia (Oikawa et al. 2019)

Muscle mass is not only critical for performance but it has also been proven to predict longevity and a longer healthspan. Loss of muscle mass is also predictive of worse recovery after injury or surgery. Our muscle tissue accounts for more than 50 percent of our body mass and is essential for metabolic health. Muscles help us control our glucose levels, use glucose as fuel, and have a role in reducing the risks of insulin resistance and type 2 diabetes. Loss of muscle mass also contributes to poor health outcomes such as fatigue, loss of function, disability, fall risk, frailty, and death.

Resistance exercise is a must for increasing our healthspan because it helps to ward off sarcopenia. A short well-balanced program consisting of calf exercises, squats, bridges, biceps curls, and shoulder exercises is critical to reverse the changes of sarcopenia and maintain our current muscle mass. We will cover how muscle mass and resistance exercises contribute to healthy aging in chapter 9.

Three ways to counteract sarcopenia

There are three areas where you have control to help counteract this age-related process: strength training, diet, and hormones.

Strength training to reduce sarcopenia.

Despite the reduction in muscle protein synthesis described above, older people can still benefit from aerobic and resistance training, so don't think your exercise is in vain (Seals et al. 1984; Frontera et al. 1988). In a study on runners, in particular, lifelong activity prevented the loss of motor units within the muscle (functional units that control contraction) in participants aged sixty-five (Power et al. 2010)! Further, some research shows that regular exercise four to five times per week can prevent the usual decline in muscle mass and strength with age (Wroblewski et al. 2011).

Diet to reduce sarcopenia

According to a study published in the journal *Current opinion in clinical nutrition and metabolic care*, an adequate amount of protein (about 25-30 grams) with each meal (for three meals per day) is essential for muscle protein synthesis as we age. Another dietary factor we must also consider is the building blocks of protein known as amino acids. Some amino acids are essential, meaning the body can't make them, so we must consume them in the diet. Aging reduces the ability of skeletal muscle "to respond to low doses of essential amino acids" (Paddon-Jones and Rasmussen 2009). However, supplementation with leucine (an essential amino acid) has been shown to significantly increase protein synthesis in the elderly (Rieu et al. 2006). We will discuss nutrition for metabolic health in more detail in chapter 6.

Hormones to reduce sarcopenia

As men and women age, there is a decrease in our sex hormones. For men, testosterone begins to decline at age thirty-five, and for women, estrogen and testosterone decline at menopause. Decreased testosterone and estrogen can lead to reductions in lean muscle mass. Unfortunately, while the solution here seems simple, hormone therapy has a few potential adverse side effects. Currently, there is work on selective androgen receptor modulators (SARMs), which bind to specific areas of androgen receptors on many cell surfaces to activate or inhibit selective functions of the steroid receptors. This selective activation/inhibition could encourage muscle growth while at the same time prevent some of the unwanted aspects of hormone therapy" (Siparsky et al. 2014). So far, the clinical trials have been promising, but there is still much research to be done on these pharmacologic options (Narayanan et al. 2008).

Hopefully, this section on sarcopenia has given you some insight and strategies to incorporate to try and delay the inevitable. Sure, we may not be hitting a new marathon personal record in our fifties or sixties, but most of us are not doomed to become frail and weak in our old age—as long as we are willing to start putting in the work now with our diet and exercise.

Insulin, blood sugar, and diabetes

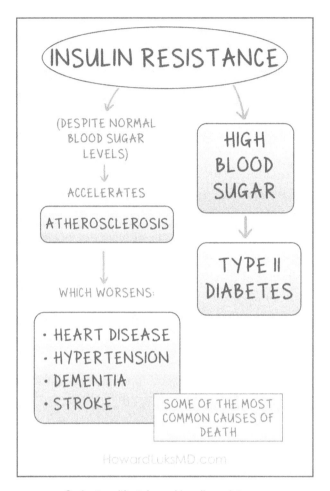

Sedentary lifestyle and insulin resistance

Nearly 50 percent of Americans have insulin resistance, which can ultimately lead to high blood sugar levels and type 2 diabetes, a pillar of metabolic syndrome. Despite normal blood sugar levels, insulin resistance can directly cause or worsen many diseases that lead to a shorter lifespan. Insulin resistance is considered pre-pre-diabetes. Your muscle cells require more insulin present to store glucose from your blood. Eventually, these cells no longer respond well to insulin, and your blood sugar starts to rise. Insulin resistance can accelerate atherosclerosis, heart disease, hypertension, dementia, and stroke (some of the most common causes of death).

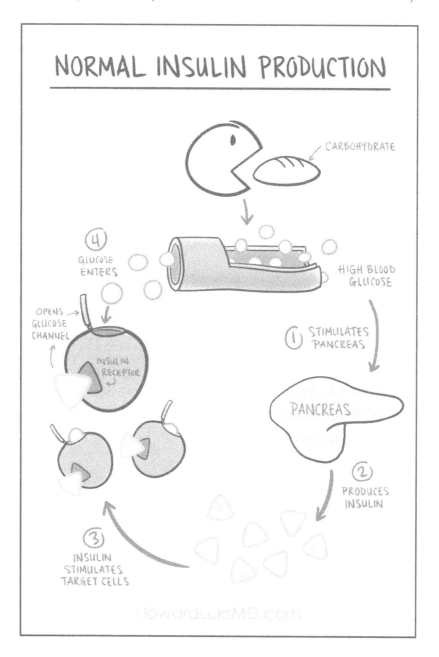

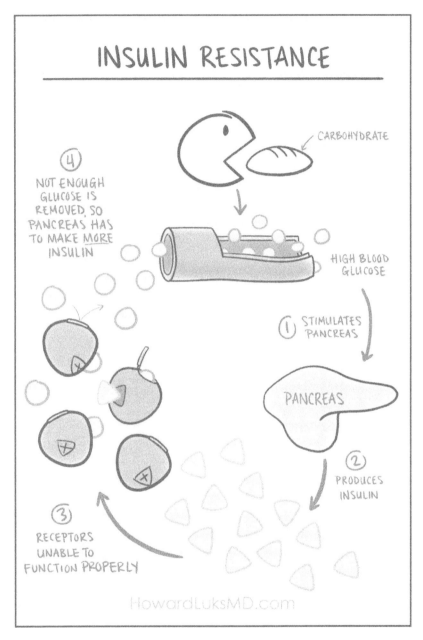

Why insulin resistance is harmful

Our blood sugar (glucose) levels must remain within a healthy range. *Insulin* is a hormone produced by the pancreas to lower the amount of glucose in the blood when it gets too high, which usually happens after eating a meal as carbohydrates are digested and absorbed. Most of your tissues require insulin to allow your cells to take glucose into them from the blood to use as an energy source.

Yes, muscles can take some glucose in without insulin, but that only occurs during exercise. If you start requiring more insulin in your body to accomplish the same amount of glucose uptake into your cells, then you have *insulin resistance.* If you have insulin-resistant tissues, your pancreas will need to make more insulin to maintain normal glucose levels. These excess levels of insulin circulating in your blood are what we refer to as *hyperinsulinemia.* One of the risks of prolonged insulin resistance is that the beta cells in your pancreas eventually stop working. When you can no longer produce enough insulin to keep your blood sugar in its normal range, your blood sugar will start to rise. Now you have type 2 diabetes. This is when your doctor might recommend that you start giving yourself daily injections of insulin.

In general, insulin resistance progresses to type 2 diabetes due to a persistent presence of excess calories, not just excess carbohydrates. Some corners of the nutritional space online talk about carbohydrates as a food group that should be avoided at all costs. That's not necessarily true. Aside from avoiding ultra-processed foods, it's the total caloric burden that you eat that matters more.

Insulin resistance that leads to an elevated Hemoglobin A1c (HbA1c) is pre-type 2 diabetes. You could call insulin resistance with normal HbA1c "pre-" pre-type 2 diabetes. These are all different manifestations of type 2 diabetes.

Do you have insulin resistance?

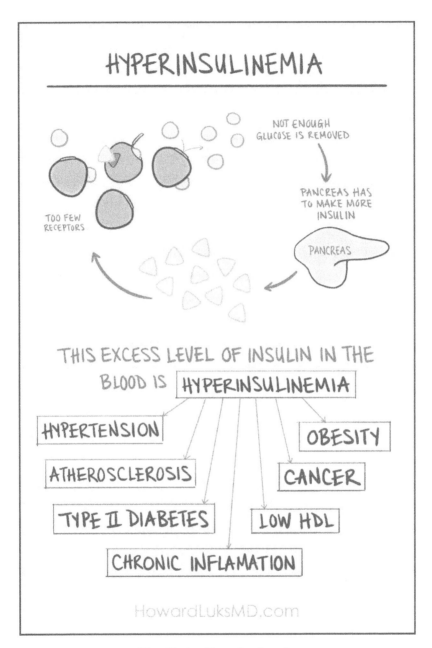

The effects of hyperinsulinemia

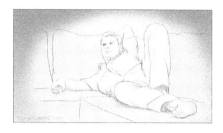

Sedentary lifestyle causes insulin resistance

The presence of insulin resistance is associated with many severe chronic diseases. People with insulin resistance do not have a typical appearance. How do you know if you have it? And how is insulin resistance treated?

Imagine if we could predict who might develop insulin resistance and type 2 diabetes long before the pancreas stops working. Imagine if we could intervene long before the progression of insulin resistance to frank type 2 diabetes and the associated chronic disease burden that comes with it.

In the earlier stages of insulin resistance, your blood glucose level might look normal on routine blood tests. Your HbA1c levels will often be in the normal range. Your fasting insulin levels might look normal, too. This is why your usual annual blood tests might not reveal the presence of insulin resistance for a decade or more. Triglyceride levels also give us a window into our metabolic health. The liver makes triglycerides from circulating carbohydrates. If your muscles aren't removing glucose from your blood due to insulin resistance, then your liver will be exposed to higher carbohydrate levels—the result being higher triglyceride levels. Therefore, high triglyceride levels are a good proxy for poor metabolic health.

Would you modify certain food groups or change your lifestyle to potentially gain back years of disease-free living? I imagine that you will answer yes to this. The issue is that we are often not told that something is wrong in the first place. We are told that our blood sugar is a little high. We are told our HbA1c levels are not quite in the type 2 diabetes range. This is unfortunate because this is precisely the point we should be alarmed and start our mitigation strategies. Most of us are not told what simple strategies we could employ to help ourselves. Knowledge is empowering. You can change your lifestyle if you know why you need to do it and how to accomplish it.

If we could intervene early in the process of insulin resistance (less insulin function per unit amount in your blood) and secondary hyperinsulinemia (too much insulin in your blood because it is not doing its job), then we theoretically could alter a very predictable path towards numerous chronic diseases associated with these processes. That would allow us to intervene while your pancreas function (insulin production) is salvageable. In turn, that might spare you a life of living with a substantial chronic disease burden and expand your healthspan.

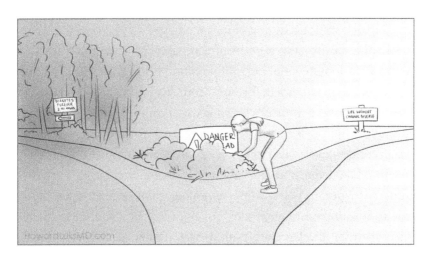

Insulin resistance is linked to high blood pressure

It is essential to know that you can have high amounts of insulin in your blood (hyperinsulinemia) and tissues that are resistant to the effects of insulin at the *pre-* pre-type 2 diabetes stage yet still have normal blood glucose levels and a normal HbA1c.

Pre-pre type 2 diabetes is the stage where you want to intervene and become more metabolically fit. Why? Because the beta cells in your pancreas are still making insulin. Years of churning out too much insulin haven't passed yet, so they're not yet tired and worn out. Once those beta cells stop working, they may never come back. That is why some people with type 2 diabetes require insulin injections.

Hyperinsulinemia also causes your kidneys to retain sodium. That means you need to keep more fluid in your blood to dilute the sodium. That is but one reason why people with diabetes often have high blood pressure (hypertension). Many diseases commonly associated with insulin resistance, such as fatty liver disease and elevated chronic inflammation, also lead to high blood pressure by stiffening the walls of your blood vessels. And as previously mentioned, both hyperinsulinemia and high blood pressure are associated with metabolic syndrome, which cuts short your healthspan.

You can think of hypertension as having a syringe full of water. You are asked to push that water through a soft, thin, flexible tube with the syringe. As you push the syringe, the tube expands and allows the water to go through easily. That is *normal* blood pressure. Now, try to push that same amount of water through a stiff tube with a thicker lining. It will be harder to push the water through the tube because the pressure in the tube will be higher. This is one reason you develop hypertension and why your heart will need to start working harder to move your blood throughout your vessels.

Insulin resistance is linked to high blood lipids (triglycerides)

Typically, after eating carbohydrates (sugars and starches), your digestive system breaks them into smaller sugars like glucose. Your muscle tissue should store those carbohydrates as glycogen.

Muscle cells require insulin to get the glucose inside the cell. There are two major storage depots for glycogen are your skeletal muscle and your liver. In the absence of insulin resistance, glucose will enter your muscle cells and be stored as glycogen. In people with insulin resistance, insulin does not function normally at the level of the skeletal muscle. So the carbohydrates you eat do not always increase muscle glycogen. They may stay and accumulate in the blood, raising your blood sugar levels. If muscle isn't forming glycogen to store the carbohydrates, the carbohydrates stay in the blood and eventually go to the liver. The liver turns those carbohydrates into triglycerides and packages them into a (very low-density lipoprotein) VLDL particle. That rise in triglycerides leads to a *decrease* in HDL production. HDL is sometimes referred to as your "good" cholesterol, so you don't want it to decrease.

Triglyceride levels correlate with longevity too. Having high triglyceride levels is as harmful to us as having high LDL cholesterol levels. This is another reason why this book will address many ways to improve your metabolic health. By improving your metabolic health, you improve your insulin resistance, which enhances your ability to store glucose as glycogen, decreasing the glucose the liver needs to contend with and lowering your triglyceride levels. It's all connected!

High insulin levels in your blood are the earliest change associated with insulin resistance. Insulin resistance leads to shunting the glucose away from muscle storage and into your liver. Your liver turns them into triglycerides and thus causes a *dyslipidemia* (an abnormal lipid pattern in your blood). Now imagine, this has been happening since you were a young twenty-something. Remember I mentioned that the longer this goes on for, or the larger the area under the curve, the worse off you'll be. The evolution of metabolic syndrome and heart disease takes place over a long period of time. Your actions in your thirties and forties can have a big impact on reducing your risk of developing metabolic diseases such as non-alcoholic fatty liver disease (NAFLD), elevated lipids, heart disease, abdominal obesity, and a markedly elevated risk of developing a heart attack, stroke, dementia, liver failure, and many cancers. If you're already in your fifties or sixties, you can certainly still make an impact on how healthful and independent your next few decades are going to be.

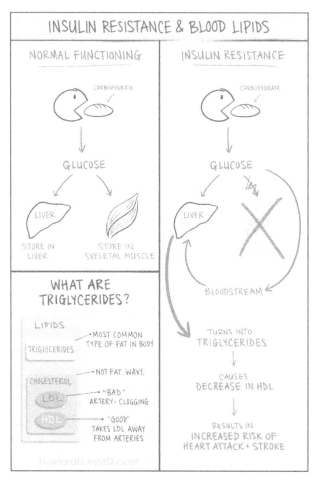

Insulin resistance impairs glycogen synthesis in
muscle (Rabøl et al. 2011)

For example, there are many reports of people reversing heart disease, fatty liver, and insulin resistance with changes in their sleep, diet, and proper exercise. So it is never too late to address your metabolic health. I also find it necessary to stress that we are not trying to treat four different diseases (insulin resistance, high blood pressure, high triglycerides, and abdominal obesity). We are treating one issue: poor metabolic health or metabolic syndrome. Treating one problem seems more manageable, no? If you address your metabolic health, you will address all the downstream issues like heart health, dementia risk, stroke risk, type 2 diabetes risk, etc.

How sugar affects your liver and increases your triglyceride levels

Lipids (fats) and sugar don't mix. Associating triglycerides with fat intake is far more logical. Quite often, there is a direct relationship between carbohydrate or glucose intake and your triglyceride levels. Therefore, let's review a bit of basic physiology and show you how sugar increases your triglyceride levels.

The liver is a highly complex organ. Sugar (glucose) is necessary to maintain life. Your brain takes up at least 25 percent of all the glucose in your body for energy use. As we just discussed, your liver and pancreas work in concert to maintain your glucose level in a tight range. If your liver has more glucose than it needs to maintain your blood glucose level, it has to do something with the excess glucose. The liver and pancreas cannot allow your blood glucose levels to rise too high. So your liver will store glucose or package a glucose load it sees coming from the digestive system after a meal or a snack. When we eat a meal with carbohydrates like sugar, the liver can do several things with it.

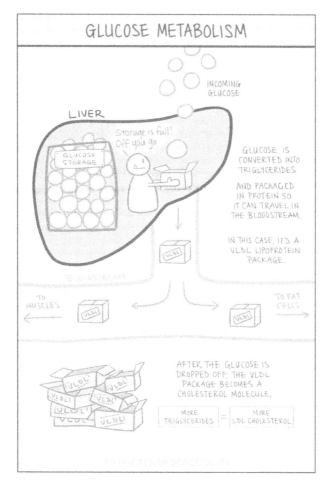

Glucose metabolism to triglyceride

Your liver can:

• Use glucose as energy.
• Store the glucose internally as glycogen (after exercise or a period of fasting).
• Convert the glucose to triglycerides, package them into a VLDL (very low-density lipoprotein) particle and send it out in the bloodstream for other tissues to use.
• Convert the glucose to fat and store it internally.

Your liver makes very low-density lipoprotein (VLDL) particles and releases them into your bloodstream. The VLDL particles mainly carry triglycerides (trigs) to your tissues. VLDL is similar to LDL cholesterol, but LDL particles mainly carry cholesterol to your tissues instead of triglycerides.

When the VLDL particle containing the triglycerides gets into the blood it can release the triglycerides at various target tissues. For example, triglycerides can be taken up by muscle and stored as intramuscular triglyceride for energy storage. They can be taken up by muscle, broken down via a process called *lipolysis*, and used for current energy needs. Triglycerides can also be taken up by the fat cells (adipose tissue) and stored for later use.

The root cause of elevated triglycerides (trigs) is often your carbohydrate (sugars and starches) intake. High triglyceride levels can have other harmful effects as well, such as causing elevated levels of smaller LDL particles which are probably worse for your heart health than larger LDL particles. Elevated triglycerides can also cause a decrease in your HDL (your "good" cholesterol). HDL (high-density lipoprotein) transports the cholesterol away from your tissues and brings it back to the liver. This is the process known as *reverse cholesterol transport*.

Triglycerides in your muscles can be used by the muscle as an energy source via a process known as *fat oxidation*. This will become important later as we discuss the role of exercise and the importance of muscle mass in chapter 9.

As you can see, glucose (sugar) and lipid (fat) metabolism are tightly linked to one another. The hallmark of impaired glucose metabolism is insulin resistance. At the cellular level, insulin resistance occurs because it becomes harder to transport the glucose into your muscle cells. Your muscles really should be considered a separate organ. They are responsible, under normal circumstances, for helping you clear the majority of glucose from your bloodstream.

In someone with insulin resistance, the ability for blood

glucose to get into the muscles is impaired, and the liver will take it up. What does the liver do with the excess glucose? It will try to store it as glycogen. If the glycogen storage areas are full, the liver will package excess carbs as triglycerides and send them out into our bloodstream. This is why elevated triglycerides are a marker of poor metabolic health. If your fasting triglyceride levels are over 100, you should consider having an oral glucose tolerance test (OGTT) because it is a more precise test for insulin resistance.

Blood tests to detect pre-type 2 diabetes

We can often predict who is at high risk for hyperinsulinemia and thus type 2 diabetes. We can tell if you are in the so-called *pre-*pre-type 2 diabetes stages. For many people, we can recognize this process very early on.

Start by taking out your last blood tests. What were your triglycerides (trigs) and your HDL (high-density lipoprotein) values? Then, divide your triglycerides by your HDL. The number you get should be less than 3.5. For example, my triglycerides were 100, and my HDL was 65. That means that my triglycerides/HDL ratio is 100/65, or about 1.5.

What if your level is above 3.5? A triglycerides/HDL ratio of 3.5 or higher provides a simple means of identifying insulin resistance and dyslipidemia and a likely increased risk for developing dementia, cardiovascular disease, etc., thus shortening your healthspan (McLaughlin et al. 2005). All of these diseases reflect the presence of a metabolic abnormality that may have existed in your body for decades. Yes, these diseases can stay relatively silent for a long time. Unfortunately, the earliest signs of atherosclerosis are now showing up in children! The sooner you start paying attention and addressing your metabolic health, the sooner you will be on the path towards wellness and hopefully a longer, healthier life.

I must state two crucial caveats about the triglycerides/HDL ratio.

1. This ratio works best if your BMI (body-mass index) is at or above 25 kg/m^2.
2. The African American population tends to have lower triglyceride levels. Therefore, different screening tools are needed, such as an oral glucose tolerance test (OGTT) (Diabetes.co.uk 2019). A normal triglycerides/HDL ratio does not rule out insulin resistance in African Americans (Sumner et al. 2005).

An oral glucose tolerance test remains the current "gold standard" to diagnose insulin resistance or hyperinsulinemia. During that test, you consume a drink with 75 grams of glucose. Then we check your glucose and insulin levels at 30-minute intervals afterward. Many people who have an oral glucose tolerance test will find that they have insulin resistance. Their glucose will be elevated above what it should be, and, more importantly, the amount of insulin in the blood will be increased.

Researchers at Yale have found evidence of insulin resistance in 30-40 percent of thin, "healthy-appearing" college student volunteers when subjected to an OGTT (Rabøl et al. 2011). This is simply a wake-up call. Over 50 percent of people might be insulin resistant. Even young sedentary folks are at risk. Speak to your doctor, look at your lab tests, and look at your belly. If you are insulin resistant, we will explore straightforward measures to address this.

What to do when you have an elevated triglycerides/HDL ratio

Eating too many ultra-processed carbohydrates can cause elevated triglycerides, and those of us with an elevated triglycerides/HDL ratio are at a higher risk for serious chronic diseases. There are two mechanisms at your disposal to decrease the amount of triglycerides you produce. First, you can reduce your consumption of ultra-processed carbohydrates (sugars) and overall calories. Second, you need to increase the number of calories you burn. You can do this.

1. Decreasing consumption of overall calories and ultra-processed carbs

We need to take in fewer calories and put fewer ultra-processed carbohydrates into our bloodstream. The less glucose your liver has to process, the fewer triglycerides there will be flowing through your blood. That will decrease the number of triglycerides in your body that your liver produces.

Remember earlier in this chapter we calculated the number of calories you need to maintain your weight? Use your number to determine the maximum calories you need to take in each day.

When it comes to carbohydrates, we're going to go into more detail on nutrition in chapter 6, but for now, know that all carbohydrates aren't bad. Keto and low-carb diets are all the rage now. Don't get lost in the weeds. You may need to get your house in order, and that takes broad, high-level changes. You can always dive deeper and refine new lifestyle changes at a later time. Everyone will not respond the same way to specialized dietary changes. A diet that works for your friends may not work for you.

Not all carbohydrates are as "harmful" as others. Elite athletes thrive on carbohydrates. Dr. Iñigo San-Millán, an incredibly well-respected researcher and sports physiologist, makes it very clear that the careers of the athletes he treats depend on very high carbohydrate diets. They do not perform well on low-carb diets. Glycogen or stored carbs are crucial to their power, performance, and endurance.

The carbohydrates we need to limit are simple, highly-processed carbohydrates such as white bread, white rice, sugar, pasta, bagels, cookies, etc. In moderation, most of us, assuming our total caloric intake is kept under control, complex carbohydrates such as natural whole grains, beans, legumes, and nuts will not cause a significantly elevated triglyceride level. Taking in complex carbohydrates leads to less rapid absorption of glucose into our bloodstream after we eat. It's the fiber that comes along with the complex carbs and berries that matters in this context. That will make it easier for our liver and muscle to handle the glucose as it emerges from the digestive system.

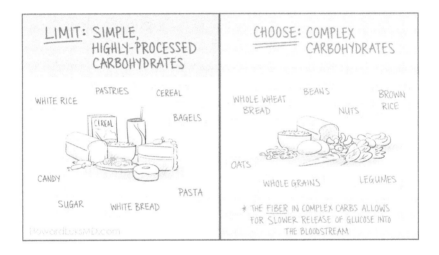

Reducing these simple carbohydrates from your diet can be a daunting issue. Some people can handle abrupt changes, many more cannot. You can simply pick one food to eliminate this week and another next week, and so on. For example, don't start your day with a bagel because white bread can be one of the worst offenders. Choose whole wheat or whole grains instead.

The main issue that drives elevated carbohydrates to be a problem is when it is present with a total caloric excess (taking in more calories than we need). It should be made perfectly clear. It's not one food group or macronutrient that is causing poor metabolic health and the obesity epidemic. It is the total number of calories we eat. Certainly, ultra-processed foods will create more fat per calorie than whole foods, but we cannot blame the entire metabolic health quagmire or obesity epidemic on carbs.

The main issue driving insulin resistance and weight gain is total caloric excess is eating too much, too often. From an evolutionary perspective, this is the only time in our history on this planet when foods have been available to us in excess and around the clock. Our bodies simply cannot process that excess number of calories properly. Insulin resistance probably developed during the time course of evolution as a means of surviving during a period of starvation. If an organism is starving, it would make sense to shunt the glucose away from the muscle and leave it circulating in our blood so that it is available for our brain. We know that starvation can cause fatty liver due to insulin resistance. Unfortunately, we are now seeing a fatty liver as a manifestation of insulin resistance in the presence of caloric excesses. So our modern eating habits have caused a well-preserved mechanism to survive a famine, and now it is working against us. Insulin resistance in the presence of excess calories will accelerate the time course of the most common diseases that lead to our demise, shortening our healthspan. Insulin resistance will accelerate the pathological changes of atherosclerosis, hypertension, fatty liver, NASH (nonalcoholic steatohepatitis), dementia, etc.

We need to look at how to deal with insulin resistance in many ways. First and foremost is to decrease our overall caloric intake. The second is to increase our exercise and muscle mass to burn more calories. The end result is healthier mitochondria which enables our muscles to take more glucose out of our bloodstream. We will discuss mitochondria later (in chapter 8), but as I've mentioned, the aerobic component of exercise that I am referring to does not need to be painful and sweaty—walking works.

2. Increasing the number of calories you burn

As you now know, the biggest sink for carbohydrate storage by far is your muscles. Muscles store carbohydrates as glucose for activity and to burn for current energy needs. So it stands to reason that the larger our muscles are, the more glucose they can hold and the more glucose they will burn for energy. How do we get larger muscles? We push or pull heavy things! Even an eighty-year-old will respond and grow more muscle from one bout of resistance exercise. Resistance exercise has also been shown to improve how your body processes and manages glucose (Dunstan et al. 2002). We will discuss resistance training and muscle strength more in chapter 9.

Exercise can increase the rate at which your muscle cells take up glucose, even in the presence of insulin resistance. This will further diminish the amount of glucose circulating around your bloodstream, leaving less excess glucose available to the liver to make triglycerides. Less glucose in your blood will decrease the signal to the pancreas beta cells to produce insulin. That reduces the insulin concentration in your blood. And the lower your insulin level, the healthier you are.

So, we know that driving glucose into our muscles can have many positive effects on our health, and the larger those muscles are, the more glucose they can dispose of and store. Therefore, it cannot be overstated how vital resistance exercise is for overall health. Larger, stronger muscles can improve your longevity and healthspan considerably.

Stronger muscles help us:

- Take up and burn more energy or calories.
- Improve our metabolic and heart health.
- Minimize our risk of falling as we age.
- Recover faster from surgery or injuries following a fall.
- Overcome the effects of sarcopenia.
- Decrease the risk of developing frailty.

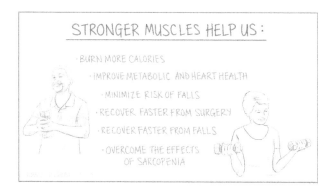

Very few people receive advice from their doctors to avoid performing resistance exercises. Talk to your doctor if you are concerned about your risk. Once your doctor confirms, you can go ahead and start, talk to a trainer or physical therapist if you need guidance. The muscles that matter most are your legs. This means exercises like squats, getting out of a chair without using your arms, calf raises, and so on are what you should be concentrating on. You can perform upper body exercises too, but you should emphasize leg exercises.

A resistance exercise program and building muscle mass is a crucial step for improving our metabolism. Aerobic exercise or increasing our net activity is also essential. Granted, you may not go and purchase running shoes and bolt out the front door, so what other strategies can you employ to increase your aerobic activity each and every day?

Making your day a little harder and your night a little easier.

Enter the concept of *making your day a little harder*. Instead of circling a parking lot to find a close spot, just head to the location that is farthest away. These extra steps add up very quickly. Don't print to the printer closest to you. Use a bathroom in another part of the building you work in. Do you need to go upstairs or downstairs? Great, take the stairs. Unless there is a medical reason not to do this, take the stairs up two flights or down three. Leave elevators for longer excursions. Have a dog? Great, they need to exercise too. Take them for a long walk. Find some friends at work who want to walk outside at lunchtime. I see this quite often; most people will not turn this request down. They are looking for someone to motivate them, too. We are going to discuss increasing fitness in more detail in chapter 7.

Another way to increase the amount of carbohydrates your body burns for energy is to sleep. Yes, sleep. If you are willing to optimize your lifestyle for longevity by addressing your diet and exercise with conscious choices, then you need to actively manage your sleep as well.

As mentioned in chapter 1, there are no physiological processes in our body or diseases that aren't harmed or worsened by a lack of proper sleep. Sleep improves how your body manages sugar by different mechanisms. The better slept and rested your brain is, the better your chances are at achieving metabolic health. The more relaxed and well-slept you are, the better your baseline glucose levels are. One night's poor sleep increases insulin resistance.

Face it, we are a chronically underslept society. We need to prioritize sleep and treat it like other important goals. Refer to chapter 5 to learn the hacks to improve your chances to get a full eight hours of sleep.

Understanding how our bodies work to influence our health is empowering. Hopefully this deep dive into metabolism helped you understand how your food intake and exercise can influence your risk of developing insulin resistance and type 2 diabetes. Combine these with making sleep a priority, and you have the power to change your risks.

Don't forget to keep your doctor in the loop, especially if you have cardiac issues or chronic disease. Speak with your doctor about changing your diet and exercise to determine your risk profile.

Let's start here!

Weight loss... Is exercise alone enough?

A friend of mine recently told me that she wasn't sure she could commit to losing weight because she didn't know if she'd have time to work out. Many campaigns from major food and drink companies say it's OK to consume their products so long as people exercise (O'Connor 2015). That's simply not true; these beverage products are insulin resistance engines. We can find the time to exercise.

Let me start by reiterating that exercise is fantastic! It provides so many physical and mental health benefits (Suzuki 2016), and you can always (yes, always) make time to fit in at least a few minutes worth in your day. But, when it comes to losing weight, exercise alone is NOT the answer (Malhotra et al. 2015)

One of the reasons your scale may not be budging (if that's one of your goals), despite your fitness regime, is that you don't burn as many calories with exercise as you think you do. One study published in *The Journal of Sports Medicine and Physical Fitness* tested normal-weight men and women who used a treadmill at the same intensity (50 percent of their VO_2 max) until they burned either 200 or 300 calories (Willbond et al. 2010). After the work-out, participants estimated how many calories they burned, then tried to eat the caloric equivalent of their exercise at a buffet. Results showed that in both the 200 and the 300 calorie conditions, participants overestimated how many calories they expended by 3-4 fold, and ate 2-3 times more calories than they expended.

"But I don't overestimate how many calories I burn because the cardio machine at my gym tells me," you might respond. Unfortunately, those machines are usually not accurate, even if you enter your gender, weight, and age. There are so many other factors to take into account, like the quality and age of the machine, your form (are you slouched over on the Stairmaster®, are you using the handlebars on the elliptical?), and your fitness level. If someone with 25 percent body fat who's never exercised before does the same treadmill run as a marathon runner with 10 percent body fat, then the person new to exercise will burn more calories. Your body adapts over time (CDC 1999) to become more efficient, so you're better off using a heart rate monitor for more accurate and personalized information (Achten and Jeukendrup 2003). We're going to talk about heart rate monitors in chapter 8.

Now, once you have a more accurate estimate of calories burned during your workout, you can think about how that translates into weight loss. Through exercise alone, you need to burn an extra 500 calories a day for one week in order to lose one pound. That's a big time commitment! Assuming you are willing to do that much exercise daily, you may run into the same problem as those study participants; you may very well eat more after a workout, preventing weight loss.

Why do we eat more after we exercise?

Although it may seem counterintuitive, a growing number of research studies suggest that this compensatory increase in food intake with exercise is not due to an increase in appetite. In fact, exercise may act on certain gut hormones to suppress your appetite (Hagobian et al. 2013; Martins et al. 2007; Schubert et al. 2014; Stensel 2010). How does this make sense? It turns out that your appetite doesn't necessarily correlate with how much you eat (Mattes 1990). People eat for a variety of reasons that are unrelated to hunger. For example, you may recall eating more when you were stressed out at work (Torres and Nowson 2007) or when you didn't get enough sleep the night before (Nedeltcheva et al. 2009).

In this case, the most common reason people increase their caloric intake after exercise is to reward themselves for their hard work. Frequently, these decisions are made subconsciously. For instance, in one study published in the journal *Marketing Letters*

(Werle et al. 2015), researchers had two groups of people take a 2-kilometer walk around a lake. One group was told the walk was exercise; the other group was a "scenic" walk. Those who exercised ate 35 percent more chocolate pudding afterward than those who went on a scenic walk.

On the other hand, sometimes people consciously increase their caloric intake after exercising because they think their bodies "need" this reward to recover. This is tricky because many products aimed at athletes, like granola bars, sports drinks, and protein smoothies, are loaded with extra sugar and calories (often more than you burned during your workout). So, if you can't make your bars or smoothies, make sure to read the nutrition labels on the products you purchase.

If you're getting discouraged because your new exercise routine hasn't resulted in any weight loss during your first month, remember that changing your eating habits is going to have a more significant and lasting effect. Losing weight is associated with a decrease in energy intake (caloric deficit). As mentioned, there's no magic to weight loss... you need a caloric deficit. Exercise has often been associated with no change in weight or a slight loss early on and then a reset of your basal metabolic rate. When your basal metabolic rate resets, it will be easier to overeat and put the weight back on. On the bright side, exercise has helped people who have already lost weight to keep it off.

The message here should be clear. Exercise is critically important to our overall health. It is one of the primary means of achieving metabolic health. But exercise alone will not result in weight loss. Exercise must be combined with a caloric deficit. So try not to fall into the post-exercise reward trap.

When it comes to hormonal control of your metabolism, the hypothalamus controls the thyroid and other organs that influence our metabolic rate. The hypothalamus can directly control how fast or slow our metabolism is. Your hypothalamus will notice the change in your activity and convince you to eat more. It will also notice that you might be eating less, and it will respond by decreasing energy expenditure. This is why weight loss is so challenging. This is also why starvation diets fail. Your hypothalamus will respond and ultimately force you to eat more, often bringing your weight back to where you started your journey—or worse. Weight loss is not easy, but it can be accomplished. This is a marathon and not a sprint. You will not find health and weight loss in a supplement bottle. Save your money. You will have success with creating a caloric deficit and walking a few times a day.

Remember the keys to metabolic health and an increase in your healthspan are:

- Create a caloric deficit, then stay lean.
- Get sleep.
- Eat real food.
- Move often, throughout the day.
- Push and pull heavy things.
- Socialize.
- Have a sense of purpose.

Take-home points

1. Your metabolic health correlates with your overall health.
2. Metabolic syndrome is a common cause of reduced healthspan, as well as longevity.
3. There are certain measurements of metabolic health, such as A1C, triglycerides, LDL, etc., and it's important to be aware of these measurements and check them annually.
4. Insulin resistance is often associated with high blood pressure, high lipids (triglycerides), type 2 diabetes. Even young people who are thin can be insulin

resistant. The sooner insulin resistance is recognized, the sooner you can take measurements to prevent chronic metabolic conditions, such as type 2 diabetes.

5. A combination of frequent movement and a well-rounded diet can often improve your metabolic health.

6. If you want to lose weight, exercise helps, but what you eat has the biggest impact on weight. You can't outrun a bad diet!

Chapter 3
DELAYING DEMENTIA

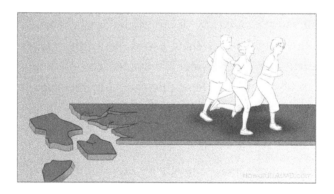

Alzheimer's disease (AD) is a devastating form of neurocognitive decline. Too many people falsely assume dementia is an inevitable part of the aging process. Alzheimer's disease is not the only form of dementia, but it is the most common. In general, *dementia* means that a person has diminished short-term memory capacity, facial identification issues, difficulty processing or encoding new memories, depression, agitation, behavioral changes, and in the end, difficulty with activities of daily living. Do not assume that dementia is simply a normal age-associated process. Your lifestyle and habits in your more youthful decades directly impacts your risk of developing dementia later in life. More than 40% of dementia cases are preventable.

What is dementia, and why is it so common?

Eighty percent of us will die from cardiovascular disease, stroke, cancer, or a progressive neurodegenerative issue such as Alzheimer's disease(AD). But it is clear that dementia scares us the most. Dementia is so common that almost everyone knows someone close to them who is suffering from Alzheimer's or other advanced forms of neurocognitive decline.

The actual number of people who die from Alzheimer's isn't known. That's because people with Alzheimer's die from something that was caused by their Alzheimer's, but Alzheimer's disease was not listed as their cause of death. For example, a person with severe Alzheimer's may not complain of pain, yet there is an obstruction in their intestine. The blockage might ultimately lead to their demise, but it was the Alzheimer's that prevented them from communicating promptly that they were in pain.

Alzheimer's disease is thought to be caused by a collection of waste products that accumulate in the brain. These include beta-amyloid plaques between nerve cells (neurons) and sticky proteins (called "tau") that form tangles inside the neurons (NIA 2017b). While you want protein to help maintain your muscles as you age, this is very different from accumulating beta-amyloid proteins in your brain. These beta-amyloid proteins are either over-produced or not cleared by the brain's microglial trash collecting system (Green n.d.). The resulting plaques and tangles start to clog critical pathways and ultimately lead to the destruction of nerve cells and the reduction in size (atrophy) of portions of the brain itself.

For decades, research has focused, and continues to focus, on the elimination of beta-amyloid and these sticky tau proteins. Unfortunately, the vast majority of all medications produced to treat Alzheimer's in its advanced form have failed. Is it perhaps because these researchers are focusing too much of their effort on treating the end result and not the actual cause(s) of Alzheimer's?

Orthopedic surgeons, Alzheimer's disease, and a goal to improve our healthspan

Nowadays, most physicians treat patients just like they did back in the 1940s and the early era of antibiotics. At that time, patients came to the office with a specific problem such as an infection. They were given a prescription for antibiotics and they were off until their next illness. We didn't know much about many disease pathways or how genetics would play a role. We certainly didn't know how many issues are tied together to interact in very complex processes within our bodies. It turns out that nearly 40 percent of new dementia cases are the result of vascular disease (disease of the body's network of vessels like arteries and veins), poorly functioning mitochondria and poor metabolic health. That means that your risk of developing dementia is similar to your risk of developing type 2 diabetes, heart disease, stroke, and fatty liver. All of these chronic diseases have similar roots in vascular and metabolic disorders. That also means that if you suffer from a metabolic disease such as type 2 diabetes you are at high risk of developing dementia. In some research circles, dementia is now thought of as type 3 diabetes.

Neurocognitive decline is often seen in association with other signs of accelerated aging. A 2019 study published in *JAMA (network open)* found that neurocognitive decline was associated with a decrease in walking speed at forty-five years of age, compared to their speed when they were younger (Rasmussen et al. 2019). This is not the only study to reveal that neurocognitive decline is linked to signs of early aging and poor overall condition.

Humans are highly complex beings. Many of the functions that our DNA codes for, and many of the interactions between our gut bacteria, liver, muscle, brain, and heart functions, have only recently become apparent. Over the next decade, researchers will have supplements or medications and targeted therapeutics that will improve our healthspan meaningfully.

As of the writing of this book (2022), we cannot prevent all cases of Alzheimer's disease. What we are learning is that we *can* reduce your risk of developing Alzheimer's in the first place. Scientists are learning how to delay its onset. Some forms of dementia may be preventable, especially those associated with vascular disease (NIA 2017a). Alzheimer's disease is often referred to as *type 3 diabetes* in some circles, but this has not been widely accepted (de la Monte and Wands 2008). Like type 2 diabetes, many cases of dementia (up to 40 percent) may turn out to be preventable. Metabolic health plays a critical role here. Diabetes (linked to metabolic syndrome) affects every tissue in the body. The brain is no different. Some researchers feel that many people suffering from Alzheimer's disease developed dementia due to an underlying issue with insulin resistance, chronic inflammation, and vascular disease.

We know that type 2 diabetes is linked to insulin resistance in your cells from caloric excess. When this happens, the cells become unable to take in the glucose (sugar) from the blood in response to the presence of insulin. Those high levels of blood glucose raise the amount of insulin the pancreas makes as it tries to help your body lower its glucose levels. After a while, the pancreas "burns out" and can no longer push out the excessive amounts of insulin your body needs to get the glucose from the blood into cells. Many researchers believe that this is a contributing mechanism to the development of Alzheimer's disease. I will go through the current strategies that are thought to adjust your risk for developing Alzheimer's disease.

Causes of Alzheimer's disease

Anyone with a brain is at risk for developing Alzheimer's disease. In its most basic form, the causes of Alzheimer's disease can be due to vascular (poor condition, diabetes), genetic, environmental (toxin), lifestyle (diet and lack of exercise), and hormonal (more common in women who are perimenopausal) issues. The potential contributors to the onset of Alzheimer's are numerous. Some of the causes are under our control. Other causes are not. There are familial or genetic forms of Alzheimer's. There are two genes (presenilin 1 and 2) that a very small percentage of people have. Carriers of presenilin 1 or 2 may develop Alzheimer's disease at a very young age.

All of us have genes that code for a protein called ApoE. But there are different variants of the ApoE gene. The protein ApoE is involved in how our body handles cholesterol and lipids. Because there are different variants of the ApoE protein, there are different ApoE phenotypes. A *phenotype* represents how your DNA code expresses itself in you as an individual. Specific ApoE protein types carry a higher risk of developing Alzheimer's disease, atherosclerosis, coronary artery disease, and stroke (Liu et al. 2013). Certain ApoE variants raise your risk for developing Alzheimer's, but some of those risks are modifiable and under your control.

Your LDL level, or a better marker of your LDL burden, ApoB (you'll recall this test from chapter 2), might be associated with a higher risk of developing dementia at a younger age (Wingo et al. 2019).

Homocysteine and other biomarkers (proteins in your blood that we can monitor) may reveal an elevated risk of developing Alzheimer's disease. Studies have shown that serum homocysteine levels are inversely related to cognitive function in patients with dementia and elevated levels are more common among people with vascular dementia (Price et al. 2018). Vitamin B deficiencies lead to elevated homocysteine levels in the blood. Vitamin B deficiencies are quite common, especially among people over sixty years of age. Decreased acidity in the stomach and a decrease in our ability to absorb Vitamin B from our intestines play a role. It appears that Vitamin B supplementation might be something important to discuss with your doctor. Many clinical trials have shown improvement in cognitive function when Vitamin B levels are normalized.

Our lifestyle choices are increasingly recognized as the most common modifiable risk factors for developing Alzheimer's disease. Depending on how you look at it, this can be good or bad. The bigger the belly, the higher the risk of developing dementia. It sounds crude, but the overall concept is that belly fat (visceral fat) is metabolically active and wreaks havoc on our metabolism. Visceral fat increases our systemic inflammation, and its presence is strongly associated with the development of heart disease, stroke, type 2 diabetes, and Alzheimer's disease.

Your overall risk of developing AD will depend on your genetic phenotype and your lifestyle choices. Your lifestyle decisions and choices can affect your risk of developing dementia dramatically.

Alzheimer's disease and metabolism

A significant number of cases of dementia can be prevented. As we discussed, our lifestyle, exercise patterns, and eating habits play a critical role. Your risk is relative to the number of years you suffer from poor metabolic health. To clarify further, like heart (cardiovascular) disease, your risk is not only dependent on your LDL or cholesterol levels today, but your risk is dependent on how many years your blood vessels have been exposed to high LDL or cholesterol levels—that is what I mean by *an area under the curve* issue.

Our metabolism plays a large role in determining our risk for the development of dementia. Typical diets and consuming energy-dense (high-calorie, low nutrition) foods in excess set us up for many chronic diseases. Our diets can trigger a chronic, long-term inflammatory process in our bodies that is a risk factor for dementia. Blood tests such as C-reactive protein (CRP), erythrocyte sedimentation rate (ESR), and fibrinogen can tell you if inflammation is present in your body. Those tests won't tell you *why* your inflammation is high, but they are a starting point.

Consuming a lot of glucose (sugar) or too many ultra-processed carbohydrates runs the risk of increasing our triglycerides over time. Triglyceride levels, as well as your LDL or ApoB levels, are considered a strong marker for cardiac disease specifically, and poor metabolic health in general. We discussed how high blood glucose levels can lead to high blood lipids in chapter 2. That chapter also discussed how your triglycerides/HDL ratio could predict your risk of developing insulin resistance which precedes a diagnosis of type 2 diabetes by years. If you have type 2 diabetes, your risk of developing dementia increases dramatically. Blood tests that reveal your triglycerides and HDL can tell you what your relative risk is. An oral glucose tolerance test (OGTT) can also tell you if you may have signs of pre-type 2 diabetes.

As researchers continue to unravel the intricacies of Alzheimer's disease and other forms of dementia, many different potential treatment modalities are emerging. Preventing or delaying the onset of Alzheimer's requires understanding the risk factors and a systematic approach towards prevention. It will involve incorporating a lot of information to determine your risk profile. We cannot change your DNA, but intense work is being done to develop substances or medications that will limit the risk brought on by your genetic code. The ApoE proteins are a target of significant spending and research right now. Being able to manipulate their expression or their downstream effects will modify our risk for heart disease, stroke and many cases of Alzheimer's dementia.

I hope that this little nudge will get you to make better lifestyle choices to diminish your risk for chronic disease.

Other tests to help stratify your risk of developing dementia

Aside from C-reactive protein (CRP), triglycerides, HDL, and an oral glucose tolerance test (OGTT), there are other biomarkers you can look at to understand your risk of developing dementia.

Homocysteine

Paying attention to your homocysteine levels appears to be highly relevant. Homocysteine levels rise in the face of vitamin B deficiencies (Price et al. 2018). Vitamin B deficiencies are surprisingly common. Homocysteine has a direct role in the cause (pathogenesis) of dementia because it can cause an increase in oxidative stress and inflammation in the brain, leading to atrophy of some areas of the brain. People with Alzheimer's disease seem to have had low folate (vitamin B9) and vitamin B12 levels preceding their neurocognitive decline. This does not appear to be an issue of reverse causation. In other words, it doesn't seem to be because people with Alzheimer's disease aren't eating enough, so their vitamin B levels are low. Overall, this means we want to keep our homocysteine levels low by ensuring we get enough B vitamins.

Uric acid

Your uric acid level also plays a role in determining your overall risk of suffering from dementia later in life. Most of us only know of uric acid as it relates to your risk of developing gout. It turns out it is far more important than that. High uric acid levels can lead to high blood pressure (hypertension), especially in younger people. Uric acid activates the renin-angiotensin system in our body, which constricts or narrows our blood vessels. The same volume of blood in a constricted space will elevate the pressure in that space. Allopurinol, which lowers your uric acid level, has been used to treat hypertension, especially in earlier decades. Hypertension is a significant risk factor for developing dementia. You should know your uric acid level, and it should be in the low-normal range, not the high-normal range (Desideri et al. 2014).

Your uric acid level is also a biomarker for how much fructose you are exposed to. High fructose corn syrup and other fructose-containing foods are not tolerated well in our bodies, especially in the presence of excess calories. High fructose exposure is a significant contributor to fatty liver and other serious metabolic issues discussed in chapter 6 on diet. Just eliminating sources of high fructose corn syrup could drop the uric acid levels in your blood.

How to reduce your risk of dementias like Alzheimer's disease

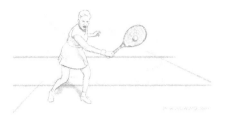

As of today, there are a few proposed mechanisms to decrease the risk of developing Alzheimer's disease. One is to reduce your uric acid levels to the low-normal range. Also, correcting vitamin B deficiencies to lower homocysteine levels may have a role in minimizing the risk of developing Alzheimer's.

The number one way to decrease your risk of developing dementia is to remain in proper metabolic health for as long as possible. Another proven intervention that lowers your risk of developing dementia is exercise. Yes, exercise.

Exercise and muscle mass dramatically affect our risk of developing many chronic diseases, dementia included. Remember, up to 40 percent or more of people with Alzheimer's have developed it because of a process similar to how we develop heart disease or type 2 diabetes. Like many other chronic diseases, exercise has dramatic effects on our DNA and our metabolism. It improves our insulin sensitivity and muscle mass and decreases our risks of frailty and falls. Insulin resistance appears to have a role in the development of Alzheimer's. And exercise reduces your risk of developing insulin resistance.

If you think of your risk of developing Alzheimer's in much the same way as your risk of developing other vascular issues such as heart (cardiac) disease and stroke, then the impetus to sleep correctly, eat real food, make your day harder, and exercise regularly hopefully grows stronger.

Exercise improves your insulin sensitivity, decreases inflammatory mediators that contribute to vascular disease, improves your cardio-respiratory status, and improves your odds of living a healthier life. Both cardio (aerobic) and resistance exercise are important. Aerobic exercise is critical because it improves your metabolic health. Muscle mass is predictive of a longer healthspan. We will talk about cardiovascular fitness and muscle strengthening in chapters 7, 8, and 9.

Alzheimer's disease researchers are studying various anti-inflammatory supplements (da Costa et al. 2019). Early studies show that curcumin may be protective, improve memory, and minimize early symptoms (Small et al. 2018). More research is needed before we can make any firm recommendations about curcumin or other supplements.

Antioxidants like omega-3 fatty acids, including DHA (docosa-hexaenoic acid), may also have a role in Alzheimer's risk reduction (Hooper et al. 2018). Some studies show some benefits and other studies that do not. Blueberries and potentially the anthocyanin found within them may hold promise as an antioxidant.

Statins may or may not have a role in risk reduction for developing Alzheimer's disease (Ramanan et al. 2018). However, in people with specific ApoE proteins, statins might make the problem worse. Science is complicated.

Vitamin B may have a role if your homocysteine levels are high. Again, no one treatment path will work for everyone. See an expert, assess your risk, and define a prevention strategy that works for you.

Creatine may have a role in improving our brain's energy systems. Energy generation via the mitochondria seems to be a final common pathway for the development of dementia. Creatine supplementation has been proven to be a safe and effective way of minimizing age-related muscle loss (Morton et al. 2015) and cognitive decline (Rawson and Venezia 2011).

Optimizing sleep is another critical factor you can address to improve your longevity, metabolic health, and reduce your risk for a number of chronic diseases. Proper sleep is an extraordinarily important part of being healthy. Proper sleep has many enemies in our busy, lit up, online, crazy world. In order to sleep well, you will need to manage stress well. There are many different sleep trackers on the market. They will give you a better understanding of how you are sleeping. Hacking your sleep cycle can significantly improve your emotional and physical health. In chapter 5 we will go over hacks for better sleep.

Again, no one dementia prevention or treatment path will work for everyone. See an expert, assess your risk, and define a prevention strategy that works for you. But make no mistake, your metabolic health is a highly important variable. It doesn't matter what supplement you take if you remain insulin resistant and at risk for type 2 diabetes. Wouldn't you exercise a little more if it decreased your risk of developing dementia by 40%?

Supplementation for cognitive improvement seen with exercise

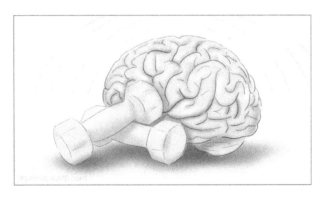

Memory improves with exercise and supplements

Both cognitive function and muscle function decline with age. *Sarcopenia* (age-related muscle loss) starts if you are older than thirty and do not regularly perform resistance exercise. As we age, we will often see an accompanying change to our cognition, memory, and recall. We are not talking about true dementia (yet), just a decline in our ability to process information and recall facts.

In a 2019 study published in *Frontiers in aging and neuroscience*, volunteers took a supplement containing 1,500 mg omega-3 PUFA (which delivered 700 mg EPA and 445 mg DHA), 30 g whey protein, 500 IU vitamin D, 2.5 g creatine, and 400 mg calcium) twice daily (Bell et al., 2019). Participants were given supplements for six weeks, followed by 12 weeks of exercise. This included whole-body resistance exercise and high-intensity exercise training. This group of volunteers was compared to a control group fed maltodextrin (a placebo supplement) and followed the same exercises. The authors found that the dietary supplement group had significant improvements in executive function, long-term memory, and overall cognitive function. They did not find the same effects in the control group, despite following the same exercise protocol. That leaves open the possibility that the aging brain requires optimal nutritional priming before the cognitive benefits of exercise are observed.

The authors also found that the improvements did not occur until nearly three months into the experiment. This brings to light that the aging brain may require longer-term nutritional support for exercise to exert its potential beneficial effects.

An earlier study published in the *European Journal of Sport Science* (Dolan et al. 2019) suggested that creatine has a protective effect on the brain's metabolism and thus cognitive function. The researchers believe that creatine helps provide energy to the brain during times of stress. These stressful events can be a traumatic brain injury or even a period of intense exercise. Dementia arises in part due to a malfunction of energy production in various parts of the brain. Whether or not creatine has a role in dementia prevention or treatment is not yet known. This particular study was not adequately powered to say that you should start taking these supplements. You should not start taking supplements unless your doctor approves them. The studies mentioned above have brought forth many more questions than they answered.

As I have alluded to before, nutrition has a role in minimizing our risk for certain chronic diseases. Exercise seems to be the best prescription to reduce the risk of suffering from chronic disease. It may prove to be true that healthy aging requires nutritional support beyond a healthy diet.

Another study evaluated previous studies to see if other forms of nutritional supplementation—or exercise plus nutritional supplementation—led to improved cognitive function and muscle performance. The authors found that supplements such as flavanols (cocoa), fish oil, extra virgin olive oil (EVOO) plus the Mediterranean diet, and others improved memory, cognition, and muscular performance.

These studies bring us one small step closer to seeing the interplay between supplementation and cognitive benefits after exercise in a healthy aging population. Many more detailed and in-depth future studies are needed.

What about brain training and medications?

In addition to the lifestyle changes listed above, go ahead and read books, do crossword puzzles, and otherwise stay mentally active.

Also, if possible, avoid certain medications such as Benadryl® and benzos (benzodiazepines).

Understanding Alzheimer's disease and your risk are technically challenging. I suggest that you visit the Alzheimer's Universe website if you are concerned about your risk of developing Alzheimer's disease (Alzheimer's Universe n.d.). Note that I am not suggesting that you start taking any of the supplements mentioned. Precision medicine (targeting unique issues because of genetic problems and other contributing factors) is the key to delaying the onset of Alzheimer's disease in at-risk people. There are nearly 15 labs across the United States which are taking intense dives into the lives of those at high risk. Those are the professionals who may be able to determine if supplements or other risk mitigation strategies are in your best interest.

Until you choose to do so, take this as another nudge to commit to exercising more. Again, sleep, a healthy diet, and exercise are the only proven ways to decrease brain beta-amyloid, improve metabolic health and adjust your risk of developing Alzheimer's disease and other contributors to a poor healthspan (Ebrahimi et al. 2017).

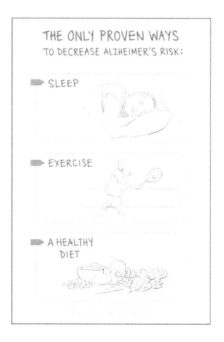

Take-home points:

1. Dementia, which includes conditions such as Alzheimer's disease, is marked by neurocognitive decline and is relatively common in aging populations.
2. Alzheimer's disease and other forms of dementia cannot be prevented, but we do know that it's possible to lower your risk of developing Alzheimer's disease.
3. Metabolic health plays a large role in one's risk of

developing dementia, and having poor metabolic health likely increases the risk of an individual developing dementia.

4. Though there isn't a singular cause of dementia, there are various biomarkers, such as uric acid levels and homocysteine levels, that should be monitored in relation to one's risk of developing dementia.

5. Additionally, there are steps people can take to decrease their risk of developing dementia. Maintaining good metabolic health by exercising, eating a healthy diet, and getting adequate amounts of sleep are all methods by which you can decrease your risk of Alzheimer's and other forms of dementia.

Chapter 4
HEART (CARDIOVASCULAR) HEALTH

It's not a secret that aerobic fitness leads to a longer life for many. Remember, my best "longevity simplified" advice to you is:

- Create a caloric deficit, then stay lean.
- Get sleep.
- Eat real food.
- Move often, throughout the day.
- Push and pull heavy things.
- Socialize.
- Have a sense of purpose.

We know that exercise improves metabolic health—which will also diminish your risk of metabolic syndrome which, again, is the combination of insulin resistance, high blood pressure, high triglycerides, and abdominal obesity. People who are poorly trained, sedentary, or those with metabolic syndrome are very poor at using fat or energy. Their mitochondria often go straight to using glucose as a fuel source as soon as you start to move. This is the picture of metabolic *in*flexibility. Our mitochondria should be using fat for energy for routine daily activities. Metabolic inflexibility is due to poor mitochondrial health which we are going to talk about in chapter 8. Metabolic inflexibility is reversible. Read on to see how this affects heart health.

I say "move often," because exercise to achieve metabolic health doesn't need to be sweaty, painful, or long and drawn out. Only 6,000 steps a day correlates with a significant decrease in all-cause mortality (death from all causes). As I've mentioned, you can't outrun a bad diet. And exercise alone doesn't ensure optimal metabolic and heart health. That's why this book includes many different aspects of lifestyle improvements that can lead to a longer lifespan, not just physical fitness.

This chapter is an example of what to look out for, whether you are sedentary, a weekend warrior, or a seasoned athlete. We will review why it is important to also consider the immense benefits of nutrition, sleep, and exercise as we pursue the goal of achieving metabolic health. The problem with heart disease is that we think we are okay because we are active and have no apparent symptoms. In other words, things seem fine... until they're not.

Heart concerns athletes should watch out for

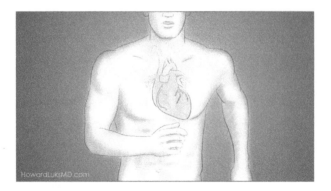

Unfortunately, tragedy can strike runners over the age of thirty-five. Because we stress our bodies, some runners are at a higher risk of dying from sudden cardiac death than many of our sedentary friends. Why is that, and what can we do to determine our risk and if lifestyle modifications or active treatment is necessary? Bear with me and read the rest of this story.

Steve was a very active sixty-year-old teacher. He recently retired and set his mind on improving his marathon times and perhaps hit a few triathlons along the way. I had run with Steve on a few races. He never faded back and never had any issues during a run until his last week with us.

Heart disease can be challenging to identify in many. A significant percent of massive, fatal heart attacks occur in people without what you might consider being obvious risk factors. Well-established risks for cardiac disease are:

- Poor sleep habits.
- Poor dietary choices.
- Smoking.
- Hypertension (high blood pressure).
- Chronic intake of NSAIDs (non-steroidal anti-inflammatory drugs).
- Your innate desire to perform better (stress).

These can all increase your risk of developing cardiac issues. Just because you run four days a week doesn't mean you should have two donuts and a latte on the way to work every day.

In retrospect, many sudden cardiac deaths are preceded by very subtle symptoms that any athlete might brush off due to a training effect, a bad meal, or a cold. For that reason, death might be the first major sign of severe atherosclerotic heart disease.

Very few of us would see a doctor with symptoms of heartburn that occurred with exercise. But you should. Very few of us would consider seeing a doctor for nausea which routinely happens on long runs. But you should. The signs of impending issues can be very subtle. The classic mainstream presentation of crushing chest pain is not as common as you think, especially in women.

Late last fall, Steve and I hit the local trails as a prelude to his final trail races for the season. Our pace and goals were normal, and neither of us was more tired than we were on any of our previous runs. One day, he became nauseous while running, but he blamed that on a work lunch before a late afternoon hill run.

Subtle clues that a cardiac event might be forthcoming:

- Fatigue—when you're more tired and not performing as well as usual—you may be short of breath with activities that were easy to achieve previously.
- Nausea—many of us bonk or crash, get side-stitches, etc. on routine hard days, but new symptoms or new-onset nausea associated with effort should trigger at least a discussion with a healthcare professional.
- Neck, chest, or left arm discomfort associated with training.

Many of us do not have a good understanding of how a heart attack occurs. Yes, you know that cholesterol builds up in your arteries or blood vessels (*atherosclerosis*). You know that can lead to a narrowing of the arterial blood supply to your heart. But sudden cardiac death doesn't occur because of slow plaque growth obliterating an artery over a long time frame.

Steve took off on his final and favorite trail run shortly after nine o'clock. By ten o'clock, he was face down in the gravel. The coroner said the cause of death was sudden cardiac death due to a massive heart attack.

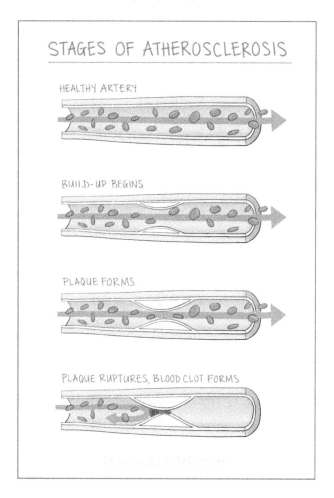

STAGES OF ATHEROSCLEROSIS

HEALTHY ARTERY

BUILD-UP BEGINS

PLAQUE FORMS

PLAQUE RUPTURES, BLOOD CLOT FORMS

The plaque that forms in your arteries isn't firmly covered like an impenetrable brick wall. If cholesterol builds up enough within a plaque, the plaque can break off, or *rupture*. When it ruptures, the inside of the plaque is exposed. We have little cells in our blood called platelets. The main job of those *platelets* is to stop us from bleeding. As they bounce through your arteries they will sense a ruptured blood vessel due to a cut. That is because of the collagen and other tissues exposed through the cut area. The platelets stop, stick to the vessel, and form a clump as more and more of them build up by sticking to each other. This gathering of platelets helps form a web to trap blood cells and eventually form a clot which stops the bleeding. This process is all well and good when it happens to a cut because it stops too much blood from being lost before the platelets form a clot.

Well, if those same platelets sense a ruptured plaque inside your heart's arteries, they will see those very same collagen structures that cause the platelets to become sticky and form a clot. As the platelets build up, your coronary artery narrows until it becomes completely blocked (occluded) as clot forms. This cuts off the essential blood flow to the part of the heart served by that artery. So sudden cardiac deaths in runners or athletes is often an "acute on chronic condition." There was an underlying abnormality—the build-up of plaque in the artery (the chronic condition), but the sudden occlusion of the vessel by a clot (the acute condition) led to Steve's death.

Remember we talked about how our metabolic health is an *area under the curve* issue? This is what we were talking about. Having our arteries subject to high LDL levels and high inflammation levels for decades is precisely what leads to the development of these plaques. They do not occur overnight. They grow silently until a critical narrowing occurs.

Those subtle symptoms or clues I mentioned earlier (fatigue, nausea, neck, chest, or arm discomfort) occurred because of the plaque buildup and the diminished blood flow to the heart. Those slight symptoms are the heart's way of telling you to pay attention to them.

Steve will be sorely missed. He was frequently the life of the party. He was always the first to the bar, the first to the dessert table, and the last to leave.

How to know if you're at risk of heart disease

What are the possible ways to determine your risk for heart disease? Do not assume that you are not at risk for heart disease because you run or exercise often. That can be a potentially fatal mistake. Too many of my runner friends think that they can have that daily cheesecake for dessert or add a bowl of their favorite ice cream on top of a warm apple pie because they run. Therein lies much of the problem with heart disease: We think we are okay because we are active and have no apparent symptoms. Heart disease is sneaky like that... we don't know we have a problem until it's often far advanced. But we can change that narrative!

Heart disease risk depends on your genetics, your Lp(a) level, your LDL level (ApoB level), and how much inflammation is present in your body. Aside from Lp(a), LDL levels themselves are not both "necessary and sufficient" to cause heart disease. It's the combination of an elevated LDL level *and* the presence of inflammation that increases your risk of heart disease.

Inflammation and high LDL levels are the key drivers of your heart disease risk. Our diet, stress levels, sleep, and family life have a lot to do with the amount of inflammation our body is subjected to. Many chronic metabolic diseases like type 2 diabetes increase our systemic inflammation. As we will discuss throughout the book, diets high in ultra-processed foods like white bread, cookies, and simple sugars can be inflammatory. Stress at work or home raises our cortisol levels and triggers a cascade of events leading to cardiac injury. Too few of us consider sleep one of the best ways to minimize stress and enable our bodies to recover (as we will discuss in chapter 5).

Identifying who is at risk for heart disease is possible, and medical intervention or lifestyle changes can stop or reverse the potentially deadly changes occurring in the walls of your arteries. Have a discussion with your doctor.

The scientific knowledge and technology to determine your risk for sudden cardiac deaths are available. Sometimes you do not even need expensive tests to determine your risk factors. Known risk factors include:

- Increasing age.
- Lack of sleep.
- Family history of cardiac issues (Lp(a)).
- Hypertension (high blood pressure).
- LDL cholesterol and your ApoB levels.
- Obesity and type 2 diabetes.
- An inflammatory diet high in ultra-processed foods and low in grains and veggies.
- Psychological and physical stress.

How heart disease evolves

What is the cause of atherosclerotic heart disease? Many people do not clearly understand how atherosclerosis forms. They think it is an unavoidable disease of adulthood. They do not understand the importance of time—and how a lifetime of exposure to cholesterol and the various lipoproteins (like LDL, low-density lipoprotein), combined with the presence of inflammation, are the driving factors that end in a heart attack decades later in life. What we eat during our formative years impacts our risk for a heart attack three to four decades later. Should we be treating LDL (and ApoB) levels earlier? Can heart disease be eradicated if we do? We will go over these exciting and vital questions in this chapter (Robinson et al. 2018).

At what age should we start addressing atherosclerotic heart disease?

If you are active online, you may have read that some strongly believe that your LDL cholesterol levels don't matter. First, that has not been proven, and that is not what the cardiology community thinks. Are you ready to roll the dice on the biggest wager of your life and not pay attention to your LDL levels? I'm not. Read on, please... this is important.

Each LDL particle is carried around in the blood by one particle of ApoB (Apolipoprotein B). Since LDL particles can be large, small, or even tiny remnants, it appears that your ApoB levels may be the more important determinant of your overall risk of atherosclerotic heart disease. That's because if you have large LDL particles, your overall LDL burden might appear high, but your particle number (which we determine by your ApoB levels) will not be large. On the contrary, if you have many smaller LDL particles, your LDL level might be normal or high-normal, but your ApoB will be high. Larger LDL particles, and thus a lower ApoB, might be more protective or might minimize your risk of developing atherosclerosis at a young age. We are not sure of this, but this appears to be the trend for now. Science evolves, all facts have a half-life, and science is complicated.

LDL particles and heart disease

LDL causes heart disease because the LDL particle in your blood can cross into the wall of the blood vessels. Once in the wall, the LDL particle can be oxidized (Ox-LDL). White blood cells called macrophages enter the wall to engulf these oxidized particles. These macrophages are now called *foam cells*. Those foam cells can die and as the process continues this causes a large plaque to form within the blood vessel walls. This plaque is made up of cholesterol crystals and all the living, and dead foam cells. That plaque initially forms and stays within the blood vessel's wall. This will stiffen the wall of the blood vessel. That in and of itself is a leading cause of high blood pressure (hypertension).

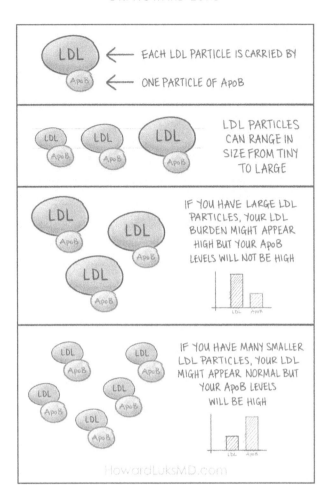

A thin layer of cells called the *endothelium* lines the inside of the blood vessel (lumen). A healthy endothelium keeps the blood in the vessel from clotting. If a plaque inside the vessel's wall becomes large enough it can rupture through the endothelial wall. Now the plaque is inside the blood vessel. That "plaque rupture" causes the blood to clot, and that will lead to a heart attack.

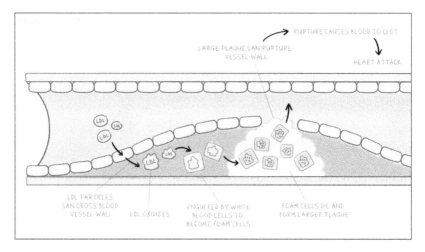

ApoB, LDL, and heart disease (Robinson et al. 2018)

Here is an important concept. Scientists find that plaque formation can start to occur in our early teens. Yes, our early teens. But we typically do not see clinically relevant events (heart attacks) until decades later. Why is that? It's because LDL-related plaques take decades to become large enough to become a clinical burden. This is what I have been referring to throughout the book as an *area under the curve* issue.

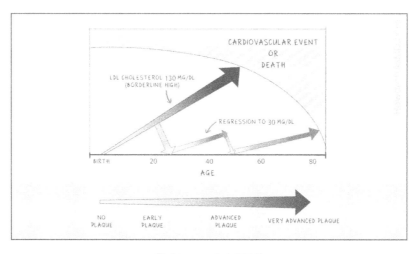

(Robinson et al. 2018)

Your risk of developing heart disease is a time-dependent issue. It is your LDL or ApoB levels multiplied by the number of decades that your blood vessel walls have been exposed to it. So if you are sixty years old, and you have had over forty years of these LDL and ApoB particles seeping into the vessel walls, you are at higher risk. This is how atherosclerotic heart disease evolves. This is why the younger we are when we sit up and pay attention to our health, the better off we are. Some plaques, if the LDL and ApoB levels are dropped low enough, will regress. They will become smaller. That happens more easily when we are young. We are never too young to pay attention to our sleep, what we eat, and how much we move.

The recommendation by the cardiology community is to decrease the LDL and ApoB burden starting at a younger age. The reasoning seems logical enough. It will take a long while until these studies are completed, so for now, keep in mind that your children do not have a free pass against an accumulated burden of LDL and ApoB related plaque. What they eat when they are young is affecting their arteries' walls now.

Aerobic fitness and living well: Let's live better lives

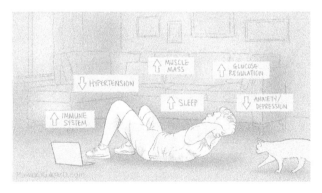

Benefits of aerobic exercise

It's not a secret that aerobic fitness is a significant contributor to a longer life. I envy those who are sharp of mind, walking under their own power and heading into their eighties with vigor and vitality. I think that our goal should be to live better and healthier throughout the years we have.

This brings up the topic of how to optimize your fitness. Do you want to optimize your fitness for longevity and healthspan, or push yourself really hard to win your next 10k? This is a personal choice. And training for the goal you choose will affect your training regimen. Later on, in chapter 8, we will dive deep into Zone 2 (aerobic) heart rate training for longevity and health.

Exercise might be the best medicine. Better stated for those of you who view exercise as painful work — *movement is our best medicine*. Evolutionarily speaking, exercise is new. The concept of exercising for health has only been around for a few decades. Humans have been moving for more than 10,000 years. We moved to forage for food, we moved to find water and to care for our young. Our bodies developed to move, a lot. Not to sit around.

When you're feeling stressed, worried, or down, go for a walk to boost your mood. Regardless of our age, we need to move often. Research shows that a single bout of exercise followed by a day on the couch doesn't improve markers of metabolic health. It's better to be active all day. For example, you can walk in the morning, park in the furthest parking spot when you go out, take the stairs whenever possible, then go for another walk after dinner. It is a common misconception that older adults should not lift weights. This is not accurate. A single bout of resistance exercise (which we're covering in chapter 9) results in net positive protein synthesis in their muscles. If done correctly, exercise will not result in harm and can hold off sarcopenia and frailty.

A critical take-home that I will explore in a different book is that you **can** exercise if you have osteoarthritis. As mentioned in chapter 1, osteoarthritis is predominantly a *biological* problem and not a *mechanical* problem. You have very little chance of making your osteoarthritis worse by exercising. The research in this area is very clear. Osteoarthritis will not progress faster because you walk, jog, lift weights or climb stairs. If you're an endurance runner, you can continue running. We know that running doesn't cause arthritis. We know that running is well-tolerated unless you stress your heart too much, so don't push too hard for too long. As with any medicine, the dose matters. Atrial fibrillation is more common in endurance athletes than in healthy matched control groups. That atrial fibrillation risk is related to the distance and pace they've run or ridden over decades. Long, slow runs or walks should be your goal. Enjoy it, soak it in, and hopefully, your metabolic health will improve, and your later years will be happier and healthier.

A recent study published in the *Journal of the American Medical Association* gives us a lot to think about (Mandsanger et al. 2018). The study, "Association of Cardiorespiratory Fitness With Long-term Mortality Among Adults Undergoing Exercise Treadmill Testing," demonstrated that the more we exercise and the more fit we are, the longer we are going to live. In this study, there was a direct correlation between fitness level and decreased risk of dying from anything—or what the scientific community calls *all-cause mortality*. Now, we all know that our risk of dying in life is 100 percent. There is no magic there, but this study is essential because we do not want to hit our later years using a walker, carrying an insulin syringe, or taking six different cardiac medications. We want to live better and remain cognitively robust.

Living healthier and perhaps longer is why I have introduced you to the concept of improving your healthspan versus your overall lifespan. By achieving metabolic health and maintaining our fitness level, we are adding years to our healthspan.

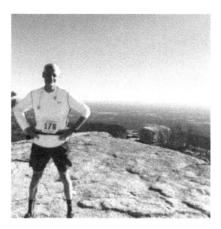

People who are more physically fit tend to live longer

For those who do not exercise, this study is sobering news. This should offer yet another reason to stand up and start walking. Perhaps don't think about it as exercise. Think about it as *movement*. Moving more is what is essential.

Just move, move often, occasionally with ferocious intent.

Most people know that a lack of exercise is bad for their health. Perhaps what they do not understand is *how* bad it is. The CDC has published data showing that only 23% of us get the recommended amount of exercise each week. The study I mentioned earlier showed that poor aerobic fitness increases your risk of dying for any reason (all-cause mortality) and was higher than the risk of dying if you were a smoker, had diabetes, or had coronary artery disease (atherosclerosis). Again, the mortality risk (risk of dying) associated with a low cardiac or aerobic fitness level is as high as the mortality risk of smoking, atherosclerosis, and diabetes.

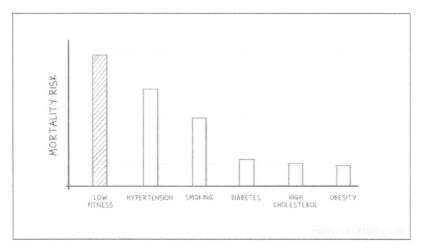

Exercise and living longer

Furthermore, this study showed that an improved level of cardiac aerobic fitness significantly decreases your all-cause mortality risk (Mandsanger et al. 2018). That means walking alone can improve your health dramatically. Perhaps we need to change the exercise narrative. Instead of asking people to "exercise" more, we should be asking people to move more.

In chapter 2, we discussed the concept of *making your day a little harder*. It can be simple. Do not park close to your destination. Choose the parking spot farthest away and walk to the entrance. Find the stairs. Do not take the elevator one or two flights up. Get up and walk around your job site or office a few times a day. Sit and stand ten times before finally sitting. Just make your day a little harder, and you will make your heart a lot happier.

It's not only your heart that benefits. An increase in aerobic fitness decreases your risk of all of the issues associated with metabolic syndrome that we discuss in this book. You get the picture. And just because you may have one of those issues that comprise metabolic syndrome is not a reason to sit still and give up. With a proper diet and exercise, you may reverse many of these health issues.

An important take-home message... While some of us may enjoy exercise, for others, exercise is viewed as painful work, and it's not enjoyable. That's why it's essential to understand that walking counts. When we use the term *exercise*, it doesn't mean that it must be sweaty and painful.

Your level of fitness matters more than the time spent exercising

More is not always better. We can become fit without having to exercise ourselves to exhaustion every day. Drinking water is healthy too, but drinking gallons a day is not. Drink to thirst. Not more than that. Whether it be exercise, medication, or water, the dose matters.

Achieving aerobic fitness will take some effort. And the method you choose will be the one you enjoy most. Walking, swimming, spinning, yoga, dance, cycling, and running all have their place... within reason. Your heart doesn't care what is causing your heart rate to rise. Any form of aerobic exercise can work. Some studies showed that tennis is one of the best exercises. Probably because it combines aerobic training and socializing. Loneliness is a grave health issue these days.

It is also of the utmost importance that you respect your body's need to recover. Recovery is a weapon for those who compete, but it's critical to rest and sleep well to achieve proper metabolic health. Your risk of a heart attack is higher, your immune system's function diminishes, and your insulin resistance increases after a poor night's sleep. Every physiological process in our body is adversely affected by a poor night's sleep. Proper sleep, hopefully eight hours per day, is optimal for most. We will discuss this in more detail in the next chapter.

Adequate nutrition is vital so your body can perform the repairs it needs following daytime activity. Just keep in mind... we want to avoid overestimating how many calories we burn in a day.

We do not want to over-indulge or reward ourselves for being more active. Yes, we want adequate nutrition to build muscle mass, but we do not want to contribute to a caloric excess for the day.

It is essential to keep in mind that people's fitness level is important, not the activity they utilize to get there. Fitness grants us a decreased risk of disease, not a specific activity—and not necessarily the total amount of time exercising. As little as 6,000 steps a day can make a difference. So, fitness appears to influence longevity and living better, but how that aerobic fitness is achieved and maintained matters too! It is possible to achieve a desired level of fitness without crushing yourself every day. Think of it as moving more and moving more often.

Perhaps not surprisingly, the authors of that same study found that the fittest among us had the lowest BMI (body-mass index) (Mandsanger et al., 2018). But, they found that the fittest had higher cholesterol and LDL readings, too. Hmmm.

As we discussed, your cholesterol number in isolation is not the best predictor of cardiac disease or heart attacks. People with normal cholesterol levels are dying of heart attacks, and people with cholesterol levels above 200mg/dl aren't. Our bodies are very complex organisms.

Your body's level of inflammation, triglycerides, small particle LDL, Lp(a), ApoB, and other parameters help us craft a better assessment of your overall metabolic stability and risk for cardiac disease. Someone with triglycerides that are through the roof but a cholesterol level of 180 probably has a higher chance of developing cardiac issues than someone with normal triglyceride levels. High triglyceride levels are associated with diseases such as metabolic syndrome, which elevates our levels of systemic inflammation.

Extreme fitness, not extreme duration, is best.

An exciting part of this study was that people with "extreme" or elite level fitness were found to have a lower chance of dying than others at a lower level of fitness (Mandsanger et al. 2018). That's interesting. Previous studies have shown a *U-shaped curve*, or *reverse J-curve*. Those who didn't exercise and those who exercised *too much* had similar chances of dying from a cardiac issue. Only those who exercised *moderately* had a lesser chance of disease and death from cardiac disease. The data on this subject is still unsettled. Three to four hours of **movement** each week is our target. Each step counts towards that goal. Even your 5-minute walk from the parking lot. Call it what you like… exercise vs. movement; the key is to move, move often and occasionally with ferocious intent.

This potential reverse J-curve issue only applies to a minimal number of people out there pounding the pavement every day or even twice a day. But it's good news because once we catch the exercise bug, we may not need to worry about the amount we exercise. Now, keep in mind that this study only discussed people's fitness level, not how they achieved that level of fitness. Participants in this study with an elite fitness level might not have been running 100 miles a week. Previous research is pretty clear in this area. People who run ultra-marathons or exercise too much seem to run into an issue of diminishing returns and possibly a problem with not being as "healthy" as they think they are.

Your aerobic or cardiac fitness matters. And it matters a lot. How you achieve that level matters for some (extreme elite athletes), but for the rest of us, it is only necessary to start to make our days a little harder. We should walk more, move more often, take the stairs, join our friends at their yoga class, and make an effort to improve our chance of living longer by simply trying to be more active each day. It works.

How much should I exercise?

Many people want to initiate an exercise program, whether it is to lose weight or simply improve their overall health. "How much should I exercise?" has become a common question I hear every week. Unfortunately, until recently, the answer has not been easy to come by. Recent research has shed some light on this topic (Arem et al. 2015; Gebel et al. 2015). The U.S. Government suggests that we exercise 20-30 minutes at a moderate intensity at least five days a week (AHA 2018). Moderate intensity means you should elevate your heart rate to 60-70 percent of your maximum heart rate (Williams 2021). Tracking your heart rate during any exercise can be very useful to monitor your intensity. The Fitbit Charge (c) is the most popular tracker for this purpose. Two recent reports have shed further light on this subject of just how much we should exercise—and what the overall benefits are.

The authors of a recent review in US News are both active physicians who conclude, based on their studies, that we do not know what might constitute "too much" exercise (Konstantinidis and Michos 2015). A certain level of exercise may be too much for some but just right for others. The possibility that exercising too much is harmful should NOT be used as an excuse not to exercise at all.

Obviously, sitting all day has been proven bad for our health. Sitting for hours on end can negate the benefits of a 30-minute run earlier in the day. Simply getting up and walking around the office for a minute every 30 minutes, or holding a walking meeting with a colleague, will do the trick.

The two studies I referenced above show:

- There is a 30% decrease in mortality if you follow the government guidelines and exercise 120 minutes a week at a moderate pace.
- There is a 19% improvement if you perform a less

vigorous physical activity, such as walking around every few hours.

- There is a 39% decrease in mortality in people who perform 1 hour of moderate-intensity exercise each day. That seems to be the maximum gain we can achieve with exercise alone.

Now, all this assumes you are healthy enough to exercise, but most of us can walk. Review your plans with your doctor and consider a tracker with a heart rate monitor. And start moving.

Hypertension

Hypertension is a true silent killer. There are no symptoms associated with hypertension until it's been present for too long. Hypertension is a leading cause of heart disease, kidney disease, stroke, dementia, and other chronic conditions.

Having your blood pressure checked once a year at your doctor's office is not enough. Your blood pressure varies throughout the day… so it needs to be assessed often. Consider obtaining a home blood pressure monitor and check your blood pressure a few times each week.

Hypertension is necessary and sufficient to cause the issues mentioned above. However, if you combine hypertension, elevated LDL, insulin resistance, and obesity, the risk of developing the conditions associated with high blood pressure rise dramatically.

Aerobic exercise, including walking, will lower your blood pressure. Aerobic exercise can have a significant impact on your blood pressure. So much so, that the decrease in your blood pressure can last for up to 24 hours. Each 1mm Hg decrease in your blood pressure significantly decreases your risk of developing issues due to hypertension.

You cannot manage what you do not measure. Please consider

purchasing a home blood pressure monitor. Use it weekly and jot those numbers down somewhere you can show your physician. That will help a lot more than the number they get when you are in their office. All too often those numbers are high due to stress.

The cardiology community has been adhering to fairly tight standards when it comes to treating hypertension. Not too long ago, a blood pressure of 130/80 might be watched. This is not the case any longer. As I mentioned, even a 1mmHg change in your long-term blood pressure can cause issues. The cardiology community is trying hard to keep your blood pressure in a tight range.

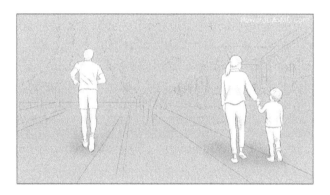

Take-home points:

1. Heart (cardiovascular) health is important no matter your age, and it's important to be aware of the symptoms (such as nausea, fatigue, pain in your neck, chest, or left arm) that may indicate that a cardiovascular event is likely to occur in the near future.
2. Various factors affect one's cardiovascular health. For example, an athlete who smokes, eats and sleeps poorly, and is chronically stressed may have poor cardiovascular health overall.

3. Poor metabolic health is linked to heart disease, and knowing your individual risk of heart disease can allow you to make changes that improve your cardiovascular health.

4. Heart disease evolves over time, which is why it is important to be aware of your risk factors, such as high LDL, at an early age so as to lower your risk of heart disease.

5. Moving often is important for people of all ages, and has been shown to decrease mortality.

Chapter 5
SLEEP!

We've now reached the next part of my best "longevity simplified" advice:

- Create a caloric deficit, then stay lean.
- Get sleep.
- Eat real food.
- Move often, throughout the day.
- Push and pull heavy things.

- Socialize.
- Have a sense of purpose.

All living beings require sleep to remain healthy. Poor sleep leads to poor health. It is time to *actively* pursue sleep, much like we actively pursue exercise. We use an alarm to wake up; we will discuss why you might want to consider an alarm to go to sleep.

Sleep is a well-preserved evolutionary process across all living beings. All mammals share the same sleep patterns. There are no physiological processes in our bodies that aren't improved by a good night's sleep. On the other hand, there are no physiological processes in our body that aren't harmed by a poor night's sleep. Consider this: If you don't eat for a day or drink water for a day, you may not feel perfect, but you don't feel awful. How do you feel after a single night of fewer than 5 hours of sleep? Pretty horrible, right? Rats that are deprived of sleep die in less than two weeks. That's sooner than if you starved them.

Physiological consequences of poor sleep:

1. Increases your blood pressure.
2. Increases the debris in your brain that leads to dementia.
3. Increases your insulin resistance and blood glucose.
4. Decreases your testosterone.
5. Decreases your immune system, specifically your natural killer cells (T-cells).
6. Increases your risk of developing atherosclerosis.
7. Decreases your ability to learn the next day.
8. Decreases your ability to store memories from the previous day
9. Reduces your ability to build new muscle protein.

The changes mentioned above can occur after just one night's poor sleep. During the early chapters of this book, we often discussed that many of the diseases we suffer from are an area under the curve issue. A lack of sleep is no different. Over a long time, the lack of proper sleep will worsen the changes in our bodies due to little exercise and poor nutrition.

Many people are very anxious about their sleep patterns. They understand the downsides associated with poor sleep, and they become so nervous about not sleeping that this can contribute to an episode of insomnia. Know that one poor night's sleep is not going to impact your health adversely. When we approach the topic of sleep, it is essential to remember that we will all struggle at times. I do too. While sleep trackers may be helpful for some, they will contribute to sleep anxiety in others, so we will not talk much about them.

Despite the importance, we remain a terribly underslept society. In this chapter, we will review why sleep is so essential and go through several steps to try and help you improve the quantity and quality of your sleep.

Why is sleep so important for longevity?

Sleep forces you to disengage from the environment. As a result, your brain and body recover and recuperate. It's far more involved than that, and we'll dive a little deeper in a moment.

When you sleep, you go through many very predictable cycles. Those cycles repeat throughout the night. During those cycles, your brain processes your short-term memory and sends those memories into long-term storage. If you learn something and take a nap, you will remember it better than if you didn't sleep until much later.

Sleep for your brain health

When it comes to dementias like Alzheimer's disease, you know they're likely to be associated with an accumulation of beta-amyloid plaques and "tangles" of tau proteins (NIA 2017b). Think of these tangles as sludge. Your brain cells (neurons) are bathed in fluid. That fluid carries away the trash and keeps your neurons healthy. If you develop a buildup of plaques, then the fluid cannot move as freely between your nerve cells. The nerve cells stop working as well, and eventually, some may die. That is why the dementia community is studying these plaques in earnest since they seem to accumulate with age. They also accumulate a lack of sleep. More than 30 percent of cases of dementia are preventable. Sleep is but one of the important strategies to minimize your risk of developing dementia.

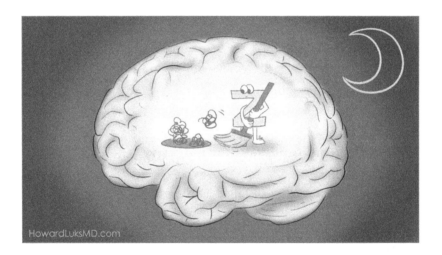

So sleep clears out your short-term memory or cache. That leaves you capable of learning something new the following day. Sleep also allows your neurons to regenerate and recharge in preparation for a new day.

It appears that we need a certain number of cycles per evening to clear the memory and to clear the tangles. Based on the length of time each cycle takes, we must have 7-8 hours of sleep. That's it. You're not unique. You don't need less sleep. Over decades, a lack of sleep worsens the progression and increases the incidence of type 2 diabetes, heart disease, hypertension, stroke, dementia, and some cancers. You may think you need less sleep than others, but your chronic sleep deficit will manifest in mid-life.

Sleep is one of the most critically essential processes for your health, longevity, and a long healthspan. Here is a comprehensive and exhaustive list of physiological processes and systems that are not affected by a lack of sleep:

1. ...

Lack of proper sleep puts your body into a pro-inflammatory state. Like I said before, there are no biological processes in our body that aren't negatively affected by a loss of sleep. Let's go over a few of the critical functions of sleep.

Sleep for your metabolism

If you want to be in top metabolic health, you need to sleep 7-8 hours per day. Sleep is essential for metabolic regulation contributing to long-term health. Glucose regulation, Hb A1C levels, insulin resistance, etc., are all affected by your sleep.

Sleep for recovery

Recovery from running, weight lifting, and illness require a lot of sleep. Our muscles need sleep to recover, our heart and lungs need sleep to recover, too. If protein is available, we will build new muscle protein at night. Our bodies heal themselves more often during sleep than when we are awake. When we are recovering from an illness, sleep is critical in the overall healing process.

Sleep for your immune system

Studies show that getting less than six hours of sleep can increase your risk of getting respiratory infections like the common cold. Sleep impacts several areas of the immune system like T-cells and cytokines. Lack of sleep reduces the number of immune cells available to attack pathogens like viruses. We need the army of white blood cells, lymphocytes, monocytes, T-cells, B-cells, natural killer cells, neutrophils, basophils, eosinophils, and cytokines to stay healthy.

For example, T-cells play a vital role in the proper function of your immune system. T-cells appear to be more active when you sleep, and their function is negatively affected by lack of sleep. Sleep doesn't seem to affect the number of T-cells you have, but it does affect the function of those cells. If you want your T-cells to find the invaders in your body... sleep.

Cytokines are another important group of chemicals for our immune system. They need to be in the right balance because too few—or too many—can be deadly. However, when your immune system functions well, you produce cytokines to tell other cells what's going on. They recruit forces to protect you. When you are sleeping, you produce cytokines to help you sleep and to help you fight off foreign invaders like viruses. Poor sleep equals poor cytokine function.

In a study, sleeping less than six hours increased the risk of respiratory infections in military recruits and the general population. In another study, sleeping less than six hours increased the likelihood of developing a cold when exposed to the virus by four to five times compared to those who slept more than six hours (Prather and Leung 2016).

Sleep for mental health

Sleep is also integral for stress regulation. Poor sleep can worsen depression and anxiety.

You need to prioritize your sleep. Make sleeping an active process.

How to improve your sleep

We face many challenges in our everyday lives, even more so during or following stressful times. It is hard to get sleep during these times; our stress levels are off the charts.

Here are 15 simple tips to allow you to sleep better, deeper, and longer:

1. Circadian rhythm: Establish a regular bedtime and waking time, so your brain gets into a rhythm. You need to stick with it. Try to go to bed at the same time and rise at the same time every day. It helps when you have a daily schedule that includes outdoor activity and daily exercise. Creating a routine is essential to help give some stability to life. Setting your circadian rhythm is crucial.

2. Daily early morning exposure to outdoor light is essential to strengthen our circadian system. In the morning, go outside and look towards (not at) the sun without glasses on. The brightness affects hormones produced in the brain. These hormones help regulate your circadian rhythm in the morning. You should try and time this sunlight exposure for the same time each day. Even if it is cloudy out, your brain will still react to the light.

3. Build a good winding down schedule. Dim the lights in your home two hours before bed (not off, just dim). We are trying to get our brains to interpret our surroundings. Just like we looked at the bright sky in the morning, we need to dim the lights in the evening.

Other tips include a hot shower or bath, stretching exercises, meditation, prayer, reading, or listening to a book or podcast. (Note: playing video games or checking social media is not winding down—it's a distraction).

4. Social media and most news sites are programmed to make you react emotionally. I have found that we need to calm our brains, especially during these trying times. Find a podcast or light-hearted comedy show to watch. Bedtime is not the best time for these activities.

5. Avoid excessive alcohol ingestion two-to-three hours before bedtime, and don't smoke or chew tobacco. Most people think that alcohol promotes sleep. That's not true. For your brain, sleep is a very active process. When we are drinking, we do not sleep well, we tend to sleep less, and the quality of our sleep is awful.

6. Avoid caffeine for 12 hours before bedtime. This includes coffee, tea, chocolate, and many sodas. Some folks are more susceptible to caffeine. Caffeine has a very long half-life (around 6 hours). Therefore, if you drink coffee in the morning, upwards of 25 percent of the caffeine is still in your system when you try to go to bed at night. Many of us become more sensitive to caffeine as we age.

7. Avoid heavy, spicy, or sugary foods 2-3 hours before bedtime. A light snack (non-sugary) before bed is acceptable. Eating protein before bed can be helpful to build muscle, but it can be filling and affect your sleep. So time any food before bedtime carefully.

8. Exercise regularly, but not right before bed. Exercise can help set your circadian rhythm (Youngstedt et al. 2019).

9. If you are in the habit of taking naps, do not exceed

25-35 minutes of daytime sleep. The best nap time is around 3:00-4:00 p.m.

10. Use comfortable, inviting bedding.

11. Find a comfortable sleep temperature setting (65-67°F is recommended) and keep the room well ventilated. Your body temperature needs to drop to help trigger sleep hormones. Some folks take a hot shower followed by a dip in a cold bath. That's brave... but it can work.

12. Block out all loud distracting noises and eliminate as much light as possible. You should tape over all the LED lights on the TV, computer screens, etc.

13. Reserve your bed for sleep and sex, avoiding its use for work or general recreation. Your brain can be trained that the bed is for sleep. If you spend too much time in your bed, your brain may not register that it's time to go to sleep.

14. Share your concerns with others. Don't bottle it up. The more stressed you are going to bed, the less the chance you will fall asleep and stay asleep.

15. You can talk to your doctor or pharmacist about sleep supplements like melatonin.

Don'ts... and bigger don'ts. These can wreck your sleep routine.

There are a few things to avoid to help improve your sleep.

1. Do not drink yourself to sleep. There's a huge difference between passing out and falling asleep. Your brain waves when you are passed out do not show that your brain is recovering at all. Drinking does not lead to a restful, restorative sleep.

2. Avoid antihistamines like Benadryl®. These medications might predispose you to develop dementia

if used too often. As with other sleep medications, they knock you out (make you unconscious). Falling asleep and being knocked out are two very different things.

3. Stay away from sleeping pills. Again, these pills do not put you to sleep. They knock you out. They do not allow your brain to go through its regular sleep cycles. You may be passed out for 8 hours, but it is not quality sleep. Besides, these medications are incredibly addictive. And some women do not metabolize them well and they will still have a sedating effect the next morning.

Sleeping properly can be quite a challenge. Our biggest issue is that sleep is viewed as a passive process for many of us, not an active process. You need to prioritize your sleep, just as you prioritize exercise and proper eating— sleep is just as important.

Take-home points:

1. Sleep is essential for your health and wellbeing, and sleeping well should be prioritized.
2. Sleep allows you to rest and lets your body recover, but it also affects your metabolism, immune system, and mental health.
3. If you want to improve your sleep, create a bedtime routine that allows you to wind down. Try to go to sleep and wake up around the same time daily, and avoid stimulating activities, such as exercising or reading the news, before you sleep.
4. What you eat and drink during the day can affect your sleep. Avoid large, carb-heavy meals and alcohol two to three hours before bedtime, and avoid caffeine 12 hours before bedtime.
5. You should avoid using antihistamines and sleeping

pills to sleep. These medications often prevent you from having a typical sleep cycle and can be addictive; sleeping pills and antihistamines can also leave you feeling groggy the following morning, making it harder to function normally.

Chapter 6
NUTRITION FOR LONGEVITY

You'll recall my best "longevity simplified" advice:

- Create a caloric deficit, then stay lean.
- Get sleep.
- Eat real food.
- Move often, throughout the day.
- Push and pull heavy things.
- Socialize.
- Have a sense of purpose.

Why is an orthopedist talking about dietary habits to improve longevity and increase healthspan? Like exercise and sleep, the foods we choose to eat will significantly affect our healthspan. It might seem like a challenge to eat well regularly, but it is a lot easier than trying to deal with the long-term consequences of a poor diet.

Your goal might be to improve your metabolic health, or it might be to improve your health and lose weight along the way. You do not have to lose weight to improve your metabolic health.

But frequently, weight loss follows when we improve our diet to improve our metabolic health.

As we discussed earlier, the only way to achieve weight loss is to achieve a caloric deficit. A caloric deficit is also referred to as a negative energy balance. Avoiding certain foods, not drinking our calories, and moderating our typical portions are key strategies.

I see many patients because of knee pain. Our weight affects how much knee pain we will experience. In addition, insulin resistance and type 2 diabetes decrease your pain sensitivity. The mechanics of walking shows that your knee is subjected to 5-7 times your body weight with each step. So, if you weigh 300 pounds, each step puts nearly 2,100 pounds of force across each knee. That's a lot of stress for our joints to handle. Eventually, that stress level on our joints can accelerate osteoarthritis and worsen inflammation. And if you are insulin resistant, you will feel more pain due to increased systemic inflammation. However, these same mechanics also means that a moderate weight loss of 20 pounds will decrease the force on your knees by up to 140 pounds. That is significant and can make your joints feel a lot better! Weight loss as a primary treatment for knee pain in people with obesity works. Achieving metabolic health will decrease your risk of developing osteoarthritis and improve the pain you experience because of arthritis.

Nutrition is important. It might surprise you to know that all I know about nutrition I learned after medical school. Schools do a poor job at educating doctors, and hence, doctors do a poor job at counseling patients about the considerable impact that their diet has on their overall health.

The number one reason we die is heart disease, which is largely preventable. Engaging my patients and readers over the years and watching many transform their lives and return to being active and healthy has been a great gift. One life changed is worth it to me. Proper nutrition, proper sleep, and exercise are crucial factors in minimizing our risk of developing heart disease.

We don't need to follow the plethora of dietary crazes we read about all day long. We can all too easily get lost down a rabbit hole. We only need to take a more active interest in what we are putting into our bodies. Simple dietary strategies can be effective:

- Consume less sugar.
- Favor unsaturated fats vs. saturated fats.
- Eat more plants.
- Avoid ultra-processed carbohydrates (think cereal, instant oatmeal, white rice).
- Include more fiber from vegetables and fruits into your body.

These are the dietary changes we need to consider adopting.

As mentioned, you cannot outrun, out-exercise, or medicate away a bad diet. Your lifestyle choices and your decisions around your sleep, diet, and exercise lay out the appropriate foundation on which you can build your longevity program. Your metabolic health matters because it affects every system in your body.

Fad diets are the rage but typically do not lead to sustained lifestyle changes. Eating real food and less of it, and getting enough fiber in your diet to support your gut are advantageous. Monitoring your LDL, homocysteine, uric acid, ALT, and other biomarkers over time gives you a snapshot into how your dietary habits shape your risk for the development of chronic disease.

Granted, no one should claim to know the ultimate diet that is right for everyone. The proper diet (for chronic disease avoidance and longevity) requires work with professionals. The appropriate diet for you might not be the same one that worked for your friend. This means that some people might respond to low-carb, while others might not. Some people might respond to intermittent fasts, while others might not. The research into intermittent feeding has not shown any significant benefits. Besides, the only way that intermittent feeding could work is if your feeding window is narrow enough that you end up with a caloric deficit. Eating meat all day or putting butter in your coffee is just an awful idea. Don't wager your life on these fads.

Whole food plant-based diets

Whole food plant-based (WFPB) diets have helped many of my patients achieve health and weight goals that have eluded them for decades. None of them initially thought that the transition to a plant-based diet would be easy. Many of the patients in our office ask for more actionable assistance. We all need help occasionally to transition to a new lifestyle, especially if it involves a significant change to our diet. This chapter will focus on easing the burden of changing our diets to improve our health, weight, and chance of living with a lower chronic disease burden.

When I work with patients to change their diet to be healthier, lose weight, avoid or prepare for surgery, a whole food plant-based (WFPB) diet is one of the options we discuss. Granted, any dietary change you choose to pursue needs to be sustainable for you. There isn't a perfect diet for everyone, despite all the noise to the contrary that you are subject to online. A WFPB diet is strongly supported in the literature to limit our risk of developing heart disease and other metabolic health-related issues. A WFPB diet can also reverse or mitigate some of the damage already caused by a lifetime exposure to a standard American diet. Switching to a WFPB can seem daunting... or downright boring. I get that. When you do a little reading about the recipes available you might change your mind. A WFPB diet is far from a life of just eating salad. There are ways to adopt a WFPB diet gradually. Some people may replace meat with fish and progressively transform to a WFPB diet.

Some people cannot imagine giving up meat. There are whole food approaches that can work for them too. All diets that focus on whole foods have a chance of helping us become leaner and healthier. Some of us may prefer to eat meat, and some may choose a low-fat, high-carbohydrate diet. Either way, achieving a negative energy balance or a caloric deficit is needed to achieve and sustain weight loss.

While WFPB diets appear to be one of the healthiest diet choices available, many people can't get past the thought of avoiding all meat. That's ok. If a WFPB diet is of interest to you, but you want to eat some animal protein, consider seafood. If you're still going to crave a steak, that's fine too; just try and have 70% of your plate covered in green leafy vegetables. A whole food diet is an important step in repairing your body's metabolism and taking the first step towards a healthier you.

Two concerns frequently arise with people who want to try a whole food plant-based diet. The first is: Where will I get my protein from? The second issue that many have is: Where will the fats come from? Finally, we will talk about different carbohydrates and which to try and avoid.

Dietary changes require that you know what your macronutrients, or *macros*, are. Unlike *micro*nutrients that we need in tiny amounts like vitamins and minerals, macronutrients include protein, carbohydrates, and fats. Whole food plant-based diets can be low-fat, high-fat (keto), high-carb, or low-carb. Again, which you pursue is up to you and your palate. This needs to be sustainable to be effective over the long term. For those looking to lose weight, a WFPB diet higher in protein, moderate in unsaturated fats, and lower in carbs (not zero carbs) can be advantageous.

If you're wondering how many meals you should have, there's nothing wrong with eating three meals a day. As with all diets, it boils down to how many calories you are taking in. The only way to lose weight is to create a caloric deficit. We will revisit this often. You need to take in fewer calories than you burn each day. There is research by Dr. Kevin Hall that clearly shows that weight loss can occur with diets low in carbs or high in carbs (Hall et al. 2021). Satiety is improved with various foods. High protein and moderate fat intake will make you feel full sooner, and that satiety lasts longer. Perhaps that's why some keto dieters have success. But satiety leads to a caloric deficit! There's no other magic involved. The only reason why intermittent feeding works is because people are in a caloric deficit with a very narrow feeding window.

How do we get enough protein on a whole food plant-based diet?

Let's cover your protein choices when you are considering moving to a whole food plant-based diet.

We need to consume enough protein to enable our bodies to manufacture muscle protein. Muscles are constantly being broken down and rebuilt. It is a delicate balance. To maintain net positive muscle protein synthesis, we need to maintain an adequate dietary protein intake.

The precise amount of protein we need to eat each day can vary. Younger folks likely need 0.8-1 gram of protein per kilogram of body weight. If you exercise heavily, you will need up to 1.5-2 grams of protein per kilogram of body weight. As we age, we need to consume more protein to minimize the risk of sarcopenia (age-related muscle loss) because our body has a harder time making enough protein to suit our needs. Therefore, even if you do not exercise, taking at least 1.5 grams of protein per kilogram of body weight is important after fifty-five. Those formulas translate into a protein intake of 60-80 grams each day for an average adult male and 50-60 grams for an average adult female (Paddon-Jones and Rasmussen 2009). That equates to 20-30 grams of protein per meal if you eat three meals per day.

A contemporary body of research shows that the timing of that protein intake isn't critical. So you do not need to bring that protein shake with you to the gym or track. You just need to include it in your day's meals and snacks.

If you are wondering, yes, you can get all your dietary protein needs from plants. There are several amino acids (the building blocks of protein) that our body cannot synthesize. They are called *essential* amino acids. Although plant protein may have some disadvantages compared to animal or whey protein, you can get all your protein needs with a whole food plant-based diet. It turns out that leucine is the most important amino acid for building new muscle protein.

The top 8 sources of protein for a whole food plant-based diet

The foods listed here can be used for meal preparation. When snacking, nuts and seeds can also provide protein.

Keep in mind what your daily protein needs are. Knowing how many meals you will be eating, you can determine how much of your protein source you need to consider using. Mix it up; these all have different textures and different tastes.

1. Tempeh (20 grams of protein/100-gram serving)

Tempeh is a traditional Indonesian product made from fermented soybeans and is very popular in Asian cuisine. It's particularly famous for being rich in probiotics—the healthy bacteria that improve and restore the gut flora, among other benefits. It can be consumed either directly or cooked to enhance its flavor and texture. I suggest cooking it. Tempeh will absorb the liquid or sauce you are cooking it in. So pick a flavor that you enjoy.

Utilizing 100 grams as a serving size, tempeh has macronutrients of 19.9 grams of protein, 11.4 grams of fat, 7.6 grams of carbs, and 195 calories.

Tempeh is also rich in riboflavin (vitamin B2) and pyridoxine (vitamin B6), as well as the minerals copper, manganese, iron, and zinc.

2. Tofu (13.3 grams of protein/100-gram serving)

Tofu comes in many different textures. Some can be cut and stir-fried. You may need to experiment with various brands and consistencies. Like tempeh, tofu will take on the taste of the liquids you cook them in. So flavor that sauce to your liking. Do not use too much oil, as tofu will soak that up too and stay a bit too mushy for my taste.

Utilizing 100 grams as a serving size, tofu has macronutrients of 13.3 grams of protein, 7 grams of fat, 0.9 grams of carbs, and 110 calories.

Tofu is also a good source of pantothenate (vitamin B5), manganese, calcium, iron, and selenium.

3. Oats (13.2 grams of protein/100-gram serving)

Steel-cut oats, the least processed form of oats, are my favorite. These are not for folks on a low-carb diet. The more the oat is processed, the more fiber content you lose. That fiber content is important, so you need to be willing to cook your oats for 15-20 minutes. There are gluten-free oat brands available if you are sensitive to gluten or have celiac disease.

Utilizing 100 grams as a serving size, oats have macronutrients of 13.2 grams of protein, 6.5 grams of fat, 57.6 grams of carbs, and 370 calories.

Oats are also a good source of fiber, thiamin (vitamin B1), pantothenate (vitamin B5), magnesium, manganese, iron, selenium, and copper.

4. Seitan (75 grams of protein/100-gram serving)

Since seitan is a product made from gluten, it should be avoided if you are sensitive to gluten. The easiest way to make seitan is to hydrate vital wheat gluten powder until it forms a dough. When cooked, seitan has a great texture which sets it apart from tofu. Seitan is one of the most protein dense plant-based foods available.

Utilizing 100 grams as a serving size, seitan has macronutrients of 75 grams of protein, 1.9 grams of fat, 13 grams of carbs, and 370 calories.

Seitan is also rich in the minerals selenium, iron, phosphorus, and copper.

5. Lupini Beans (26 grams of protein/cup)

Lupini beans are a fantastic protein source for people on a low-carb, high-fat, plant-based diet. They contain a lot of protein and fiber and very few carbs.

Utilizing 1 cup as a serving size, lupini beans have macronutrients of 26 grams of protein, 5 grams of fat, 16 grams of carbs, and 198 calories.

Lupini beans contain generous amounts of fiber, vitamin A, folate (vitamin B9), magnesium, manganese, copper, phosphorus, potassium, and zinc.

6. Edamame (12.4 grams of protein/100-gram serving)

Edamame are immature soybeans. They make for a quick, great snack and can be used as a protein source for meals.

Utilizing 100 grams as a serving size, edamame has macronutrients of 12.4 grams of protein, 6.4 grams of fat, 6.7 grams of carbs, and 141 calories.

Edamame also contains omega-6 fatty acids, thiamine (vitamin B1), folate (vitamin B9), vitamin C, iron, and potassium.

7. Lentils (9 grams of protein/100-gram serving)

Lentils are too high in carbs for people on keto or low-carb high-fat diets. Lentils should be a staple in a whole food plant-based *non-keto* diet. There are different colors and types of lentils. Each one has a unique flavor and purpose.

Utilizing 100 grams as a serving size, lentils have macronutrients of 9 grams of protein, 0.4 grams of fat, 14.3 grams of carbs, and 116 calories.

Lentils are rich in fiber, thiamine (vitamin B1), pantothenate (vitamin B5), folate (vitamin B9), iron, copper, and manganese.

8. Quinoa (8 grams of protein/cup)

Quinoa is one of the most popular seed sources of protein in the world. Quinoa is gluten-free, and it is very high in soluble fiber.

Utilizing 1 cup as a serving size, quinoa has macronutrients of 8 grams of protein, 4 grams of fat, 40 grams of carbs, and 222 calories.

Quinoa contains fiber, thiamine (vitamin B1), folate (vitamin B9), magnesium, manganese, copper, and iron.

Fiber!

There is no disputing the overall benefits of a diet high in fiber. The fiber in our diet comes from plants and grains. We do not get fiber from animal protein sources.

Fiber is found in soluble and insoluble forms. The insoluble form (e.g., Psyllium husk [Metaucil]) is helpful for those trying to regulate their bowel movements and those who suffer from constipation.

Most of the benefits of a diet high in fiber come from soluble fiber. To better understand why we need to take a moment and discuss our gut microbiome. In our gut, we have trillions of bacteria. There are many different species of bacteria present in our microbiome. Some can be harmful to us, and many are beneficial.

Our gut has a tremendous role in our overall health. Our gut is not a passive digestive machine to break down and absorb the foods we eat. For example, 75% of the dopamine and serotonin that nerve cells in the brain use to communicate comes from the gut. The wonders of the gut and its role in our overall health are a focus of significant study.

When we eat, we are feeding our microbiome. Those bacteria break down the foods we eat, and we absorb their breakdown products. Many of these breakdown products the bacteria leave behind are very healthy for us. If we eat well we have a diverse and healthy microbiome. Most people who eat a standard American diet have a far less diverse microbiome. This lack of diversity puts us at risk for various diseases. Stool transplants—basically the transfer of bacteria from the gut to someone else—have been able to treat obesity and other disease states. This is another area of study to keep a close eye on. Building back the diversity of our microbiome is accomplished with the appropriate changes to the foods we choose to eat.

When we consume soluble fiber, it forms a thick slime on the inside of our gut walls. This slows our absorption of glucose, which helps our body manage a glucose load. The true benefit of soluble fiber comes from our microbiome. Our gut cannot break down or metabolize the soluble fiber. The bacteria in our gut ingest the fiber and release short-chain fatty acids in response. We then absorb those fatty acids. Short-chain fatty acids improve the health of our gut, heart, blood vessels, and brain. Short-chain fatty acids decrease the risk of colon cancer and reduce our risk of developing heart disease and other chronic diseases.

There are many different types of soluble fiber. Each plant species has a slightly different soluble fiber. The beneficial bacteria in our gut become more plentiful on a high-fiber diet. We improve our bacterial diversity when we increase the variety of the plants that we eat.

The loss of microbial diversity in our gut increases the risk of us developing obesity and many different disease states. Maintaining a healthy gut is just as important as:

- Proper sleep.
- Proper nutrition.
- Getting enough exercise.

How do we get enough healthy fats on a whole foods plant-based diet?

Since the 1980s, we have been barraged with the notion that fat is bad—all fat, period. The food industry took notice and took advantage. Everything became low-fat, but they substituted ultra-processed carbohydrates for the fat they had removed from the foods. It's now become apparent, and more research proves this everyday, that not all carbohydrates are good and not all fats are bad.

Since the low-fat craze began, several things have happened:

1. Obesity rates have skyrocketed.
2. The incidence of type 2 diabetes has increased.
3. Systemic inflammation within our body has become the norm.

The obesity epidemic and surge in metabolic diseases like type 2 diabetes cannot be blamed on carbohydrates alone. The low fat craze initiated the changes that led to a lot of the manipulation of the foods that are available to us in the supermarket. Many of our foods are now ultra-processed. They are less satiating. Ultra-processed foods lead to more weight gain than an equally weighted portion of whole foods. This entire process has led to a significant rise in the overall calories we eat. The dramatic rise in metabolic disease and obesity is now an issue of caloric excess. Yes, some genetic processes are involved, but we were not meant to have calorie-dense foods available 24 hours, 7 days a week.

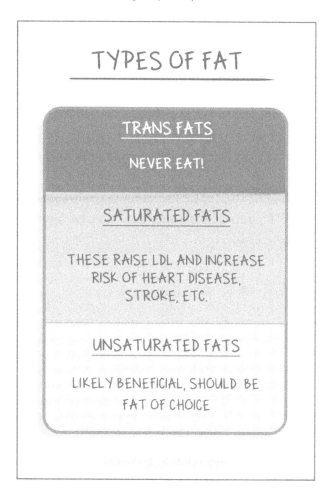

Eating fat is not always bad for you.

There are many ways to get healthy, essential fats into your diet on a whole food plant-based diet. It turns out that eating some types of fat is not bad for you, and some forms of fat are likely protective and beneficial (Time 2014).

Eating mono- and poly-**unsaturated fats** might lower our risk of heart disease and diabetes. However, we cannot make formal or strict recommendations about whether or not certain fats should be eaten to minimize our risk of developing heart disease, obesity, and diabetes. But the picture is becoming clearer:

- Avoid all trans fats. End of story.
- Saturated fats. The cardiology data is clear, saturated fats raise LDL(ApoB), and that, in combination with inflammation, will increase our risk of heart disease, stroke, etc.
- Unsaturated fats will likely be proven to be beneficial for us and, until proven otherwise, should be utilized as the fat of choice when preparing our meals.
- The biggest issue with fats is that they are calorie-dense. That means that they have a lot of calories associated with them.

Carbohydrates

High fat diets might not be in our best interest, but fat as a whole is probably not the issue that ultra-processed carbohydrates are. Ultra-processed carbohydrates (sugars) can be found in very high amounts in many foods we eat. Looking at the ingredient list, you might be fooled into thinking otherwise. "Big food" has found ways to hide sugar in our foods by changing the names of the ingredients or stating it is organic or raw. They are still processed sugars. As we have said throughout the book, It is not one food macro responsible for the obesity epidemic. The issue that leads most of us to gain weight is that we consume too many calories as a whole, as we discussed in chapter 2.

Watch the ultra-processed carbohydrate content in your foods. Do not be so afraid of some of the fats you are eating. Packages and labels of "big food" products can be very misleading. "Low-fat" does necessarily mean it is healthy because the other ingredients you may not be able to pronounce are forms of sugar and ultra-processed carbohydrates that are no better for you.

Please don't take home the wrong message. A poor diet doesn't come from eating too much of one food group versus the other. It comes from our total caloric intake—we eat too much.

We can achieve metabolic health with low-carb, high-fat, or high-carb diets. It's the overall caloric burden that you eat that matters most of all.

Ultra-processed carbohydrates are not OK

Carbohydrates are getting a bad rap. Some of them should. Ultra-processed carbohydrates are proven to lead to more fat gains when compared to isocaloric complex carbohydrate intake. That means that after eating 200 kilocalories of ultra-processed carbs vs. a *complex* carb, like beans, you will gain more fat mass due to the processing of the foods.

Carbohydrates that are OK

OK, so what are "good" carbohydrates?

Good carbohydrates are *complex* carbs (think of plants such as nuts, vegetables, and fruits). Examples include: beans, oatmeal, walnuts, apples, bananas, and carrots.

Complex carbohydrates take longer for your body to metabolize. This means they have a lower glycemic index because of the slower absorption in your intestines. Complex carbs do not result in an insulin rush. That is attributable to the fiber which comes along with eating whole foods. The fiber in fruit binds the sugars in fruit, so they do not have the same effect as a bowl of cereal.

Elimination diets aren't necessary, nor are they likely to be proven to be healthy in the long run. Lifestyle changes are required. Lifestyle changes will get us to where we need to be. Lifestyle changes are sustainable. I am not saying this is easy—quite the contrary, I have witnessed the struggle every day in my office.

Metabolic health and weight loss are achieved through a caloric deficit until you have reached your ideal weight. Metabolic health alone is achievable even if you hold on to excess weight.

The key is not to overeat and to focus on real foods. The food groups or macronutrients you choose to achieve that goal are less relevant. It is the total caloric intake that matters most.

Plants such as nuts, vegetables, and fruits are a very big part of the answer for a longer healthspan. It's not an easy change—but look at all the people around you. Who would enjoy having you around a bit longer than your current lifestyle will support? Making those lifestyle changes to increase your healthspan is worth it. You're worth it.

Are sports drinks and juice potentially harmful to our health?

Far too many people still believe that a glass of orange juice in the morning is the right thing to do. Similarly, far too many still believe that downing a sports drink during running, tennis, and soccer is necessary. Let's discuss why juices, sports drinks, and other sugary beverages are potentially harmful to our health. Again, obesity is due to a caloric excess. Children in the US are starting to suffer from obesity, type 2 diabetes, hypertension, and heart disease. Sports drinks and juices add to calories and are often not necessary. In general, we should not drink our calories. Some athletic events require sugar to replace our losses. But the vast majority of us only require water to replace our fluid loss when we exercise.

It has long been suspected that fructose (a type of sugar) is capable of causing significant harm when ingested in powder and liquid forms such as juices and sports drinks. The food industry's development of high fructose corn syrup only made this worse. The human body does not need fructose. It is not an essential sugar necessary for us to survive or thrive.

Over the last few years, many scientists have theorized that fructose might be one of the leading causes of diseases such as cardiac disease, insulin resistance, elevated LDL, elevated triglycerides, fatty liver, and the metabolic syndrome seen in adults and children throughout the US. These are harmful diseases that could significantly shorten our lifespan and healthspan.

The history of fructose and why it is in our diet

Fructose was discovered in the late 1800s. Fructose has been used as the primary sweetener of foods because it is cheap to manufacture. Fructose is twice as sweet as sucrose (table sugar), making food more palatable, and arguably more addictive. The food industry uses various forms of fructose. A widespread form is high fructose corn syrup (HFCS).

Recent data from the National Health and Nutrition Examination Survey (NHANES) shows that nearly half of all Americans consume high fructose corn syrup in a sugary beverage every day. Many will consume between 200-500 calories per day of fructose, and there are 15 calories in a single teaspoon! Fructose is considered an "added" sugar when you read a food label. Both the US Recommended Daily Allowance (RDA) and the World Health Organization (WHO) suggest significantly limiting "added" sugar in our diets. The daily recommendations are 100 calories per day (US RDA) or no more than 10 percent of total calories (WHO) of sugar. If there wasn't tremendous political pressure put on both the US RDA and the WHO, I imagine those recommended numbers would drop much further.

First, some useful definitions.

Fructose. A five-carbon ring sugar found in fruit. Human evolution gave us a way to get rid of it, but evolution has declared that fructose is not a necessary part of the human diet. We need glucose, vitamins, minerals, protein, and fats to survive.

NAFLD: Non-alcoholic fatty liver is thought to affect nearly 40 percent of Americans. It is characterized by excess fat accumulation in the liver. It is more commonly seen in adults and children with obesity. NAFLD is frequently seen in association with type 2 diabetes as well as lipid-related issues such as an elevated LDL and triglycerides. NAFLD is not as dangerous as NASH.

NASH: In a certain percentage of patients with NAFLD, they will also go on to develop inflammation within the liver. This inflammation, called non-alcoholic steatohepatitis, scars the liver and in time may lead to cirrhosis. Many patients with end-stage cirrhosis might go on to require a liver transplant. NASH is far more severe than NAFLD.

Microbiome: The microbiome is composed of trillions of bacteria within your gut. It has become abundantly clear that these bacteria play a significant role in obesity, depression, certain diseases, and how we metabolize many of the foods we eat.

Why is fructose bad for us?

Excess fructose can cause fatty liver and increases in triglycerides, uric acid, and heart (cardiac) disease.

What happens to fructose when you eat it? You may recall earlier in chapter 2 when we reviewed how the liver metabolizes glucose. Fructose is different. Uric acid is produced during the metabolism of fructose. That is why we can potentially use your uric acid level as a biomarker for the amount of fructose you ingest. If you suffer from gout, this increase could initiate a gout attack.

Glucose typically follows a pathway resulting in the production of glycogen, which is how our body stores energy. On the other hand, the metabolism of fructose often ends in the production of fatty acids. That is one mechanism of how fructose increases the amount of fat in your liver. That can lead to a fatty liver or non-alcoholic fatty liver disease (NAFLD).

The liver will try its hardest to get rid of those extra fats. It will package the fat into a particle known as a very-low-density lipoprotein (VLDL). Those VLDLs are full of triglycerides from your liver.

During their trip through your bloodstream, those lipids can find their way into your blood vessel walls. When combined with inflammation, which is produced by high sugar loads, the combination can cause atherosclerosis. That is how fructose can cause fatty liver, increased triglycerides, increased uric acid, and cardiac disease.

A recent study published in the *Journal of the American Medical Association* showed that a single 12-ounce glass of juice or a sugary beverage was associated with an 11 percent increase in all-cause mortality (death due to any reason). Two servings a day increased that risk to 24 percent (Collin et al. 2019).

The bottom line on fructose

Fructose is a very commonly used sweetener. You have no biological or nutritional need for it. Excess fructose appears capable of causing disease in humans and animals. It is a common misconception that sports or vitamin drinks are healthy. They are not. They are full of fructose and other forms of sugar. Most exercise does not require immediate replenishment of your energy expenditure. That means that if you go for a 10-mile run, you can drink water and wait until you get home so you can make yourself a much healthier meal. For marathon training and runs longer than 15 miles, you may need minerals and calories as well. But if you are not one of those 0.1 percent of people running that far, you do not need these sugar-laden sports drinks, sodas, and iced teas.

The same goes for our children on the ballfield. They do not require Gatorade® or other sports drinks. They should be mainly drinking water. Electrolyte powders are ok for hot days or very long games.

Water should be the primary beverage we choose throughout the day. The food industry will try very hard to convince you that the opposite is true. They are not vested in your health and well-being. Prioritize your health. Prioritize your health long into the future. Water should be your first drink of choice.

Transitioning to a whole food plant-based diet

Transitioning to a whole food plant-based diet is not easy, but the effort is worth it. As you may recall, your metabolic health affects your joints, tendons, and overall healthspan. A whole food plant-based diet has helped many achieve weight loss and significant improvement in their metabolic health. As you may recall, your metabolic health affects your joints, tendons, and overall healthspan. These changes may have even allowed some to put off their knee replacement surgery. For others, being in better health lessens the risks associated with surgery and eases their recovery.

When it comes to achieving metabolic health and increasing your healthspan—it's not just about sugar or ultra-processed carbohydrates. It's our total calorie intake, hopefully, with less saturated fats, that matters.

For those who are interested in the science and health benefits associated with a WFPB diet, I would strongly suggest following Dr. Danielle Belardo. She is a cardiologist and WFPB advocate, she shares a wealth of experience from the office and from her kitchen.

Take-home points:

1. A whole-food plant-based (WFPB) diet has many health benefits and can increase your healthspan and improve your metabolic health.
2. There are various whole food plant-based sources of protein available, meaning you don't have to eat meat to receive adequate amounts of protein.
3. Whole food plant-based diets are often high in fiber, and fiber is often essential to good gut health. Like

your metabolic health, your gut health can have a
major effect on your body.

4. When it comes to fats, trans fats should be avoided and
saturated fats should be limited. Unsaturated fats have
been shown to benefit our health.

5. Carbohydrates aren't inherently unhealthy or bad for
you, but ultra-processed forms of carbohydrates, such
as sports drinks or foods with large amounts of
fructose, can negatively impact your metabolic health
and should be avoided.

Chapter 7
THE BENEFITS OF EXERCISE

It is challenging for us who often exercise to understand why exercise is so challenging for most people to adopt. I think medicine does a poor job explaining what an exercise program for most people might look like. This chapter will review how to craft an exercise program and its benefits. Those who already enjoy exercising and those interested in starting an exercise program will both find topics of interest in this chapter.

It is important to understand; an exercise program doesn't need to involve pain, sweat, and hours leaning over on an elliptical machine. In the end, the key to an exercise program is to move— and move often. Perhaps that movement might, on occasion, involve ferocious intent.

No matter the reason, studies are clear that movement is beneficial for us, as inactivity triggers many metabolic processes that have harmful effects on our health. As we have discussed throughout the book, poor metabolic health is often the root cause of many chronic diseases. The root cause of poor metabolic health are poorly functioning mitochondria. A good night's sleep improves mitochondrial function, but an exercise program is needed to increase the number of mitochondria and improve how well they function. Thus, it is key to move and move often to improve our metabolic health.

Pursuing a longer "healthspan," the period of time that you are cognitively intact and physically able, does not need to be complicated. When starting a new exercise program, inevitably, it will be viewed as work. For many, that will be unpleasant enough to cause most to stop exercising. Let's face it; change is hard. However, habits, once formed, are easy to maintain.

What does work is seeing the benefits... once it becomes routine and people feel better in general or feel better for accomplishing something, it often sticks.

Do you find it hard to get out of a chair? Climb stairs? Walk up a hill? This doesn't have to be your norm.

Failure to adopt a new exercise program is often associated with too lofty and unrealistic goals. Let's change that! How can you approach this in a way that will make your lifestyle changes stick? This chapter will help you stop sitting, start moving, and stay active.

Activity goals

The U.S. Government recommends 30 minutes of "exercise" 5 days a week. There's a reason that less than 25 percent of people achieve that (CDC 2021). It's hard. At least it seems so! Studies show that walking around the office or standing at your desk and doing calf raises every 30 minutes can lower your blood pressure, minimize blood sugar spikes, and provide a sound start towards your goals of maximizing your healthspan.

Setting goals is difficult, and if they're too lofty or long-term, they're often a recipe for failure. Most of us stress about big projects because we look too far off in the distance at the finish line, unsure how to get there.

Enter the concept of *chunks*: little pieces. Break up your goals into bite-size chunks. That way realizing the goal isn't someday way off in the future; it is a week from now. Make the goal achievable. For example, the thought of losing 60 pounds seems daunting... but do you think you can lose 1 pound per week?

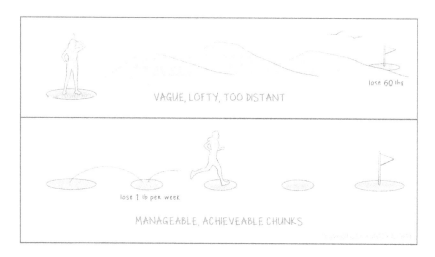

Your goal at the beginning of any journey towards a healthier you needs to be achievable. You may remember in chapter 2 where we introduced the concept of *making your day a little harder*. This was started by a brilliant family practice doctor in Canada— kudos to Dr. Mike Evans. The concept is simple. At home, move your printer far away from your computer. Park in a spot at the back of the lot. Walk those two flights of stairs up or five flights down (no elevators). Ever have a walking meeting? Try one. Ever go out for a walk with young children? They'll love the time alone with you... and you'll be amazed what they share when both of you aren't buried in your iPad or phone.

Another reason why it is best to have many little bits of activity throughout the day is because the longer you're sedentary, the more physical benefits you lose. For example, if you sit on your Peloton® for an hour in the morning, then sit all day at work and do not walk around, then you lose some of the physical benefits of the ride in the morning.

Ready to move beyond simple, science-proven lesser activity goals and start a physical fitness program? Great! We're going to cover exactly how to do this using the concept of "base building" in chapter 8.

Exercise benefits for your whole health

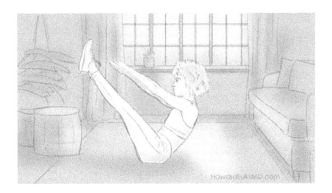

Far too many people are not exercising at the very time it could have its greatest payoff. Failing to exercise when you feel anxious, sad, and lonely is like not taking an Aspirin® when you have a terrible headache. Perhaps if we understood exactly why exercise is so important, it would motivate us to take it as seriously as we should.

During times of stress or uncertainty, we easily adopt unhealthy sedentary habits even though it is at these times when it is more critical than ever to prioritize your health and well-being. However, with a little effort, we can create new, healthier habits.

Exercise is the best medicine for your physical and emotional well-being. Exercise impacts our weight, our glucose metabolism, our sleep, blood pressure, and the function of our immune system. How does exercise do this?

Exercise for your longevity

The amount of muscle you have (your overall muscle mass) contributes significantly to your longevity. Muscles are highly metabolic tissues. They burn fat and blood sugar (glucose) and are our most important contributors to glucose regulation. Your legs have the largest and most powerful muscle groups in your body. When exercising you should prioritize leg exercises to get the most mass and metabolic effects for your effort.

If you are trying to improve your chances of having fewer issues with recovering after being sick, muscle mass is important to prioritize. Studies have shown that new muscle protein is increased after just one set of resistance exercise. So there is no excuse for not starting today. Just take it slow, as you don't want to be too sore.

Don't have any equipment or weights at home? That's fine. It is possible to craft an exercise program based only on bodyweight exercises. You can maintain your current muscle mass, and build new muscle mass without wasting one dollar on any special equipment.

There are many platforms available to help you. Fitness Blender is but one. They offer plenty of bodyweight workout programs. Paid apps such as future.co can also be very useful and motivational. A local trainer can advise you on a program based on your own needs and goals. A few caveats. Start off slowly. You shouldn't be in pain for days after a workout. Don't do it too often. Remember, we need to give our body a chance to recover. You do not need to exercise to exhaustion. You will build new muscle mass without having to push out that last rep with all you have left in the tank. And most important. Talk to your doctor before initiating an exercise program.

Exercise for your metabolic health

Metabolism is how your body uses food (fat and glucose) to produce energy. Our bodies prefer to utilize fat for energy production, but poor metabolic health preferentially uses more glucose instead. People who burn more glucose for energy to sustain simple activities of daily living have poor metabolic health due to mitochondrial inflexibility, as we will discuss in chapter 8. People who are metabolically fit will burn fat until exercise increases the demand for energy over and beyond what fat burning alone can supply.

Poor mitochondrial function is the root cause of many metabolic diseases such as type 2 diabetes. Exercise will improve the number of mitochondria and improve how efficiently they process fat and glucose for energy. We will cover this in more detail in Chapter 8.

Insulin resistance and type 2 diabetes alter your ability to regulate your blood sugar (glucose). Exercise helps your muscles become more sensitive to the effects of insulin (the hormone that helps regulate blood sugar), so they can overcome their resistance. The more you exercise, the more sensitive to insulin your muscles become.

Type 2 diabetes is often associated with other metabolic diseases such as fatty liver, abdominal obesity, and metabolic syndrome. These conditions are both caused by and lead to further chronic inflammation. The chronic inflammation associated with diabetes can be controlled by better regulation of your glucose metabolism.

In addition, during exercise, you will burn more calories and thus more glucose. As long as you don't reward yourself with a sweet treat after your routine, you will diminish your overall glucose stores in your body. This will improve your type 2 diabetes, fatty liver, hypertension, and metabolic syndrome.

Exercise for better sleep

Remember from chapter 5, there are no biological processes in our body that aren't negatively affected by a loss of sleep. Exercise improves your chance of getting a good night's sleep. Just don't exercise too close to your bedtime. Your body temperature needs to decrease to allow you to sleep, and exercise will raise your core temperature. Try to exercise at least two hours before going to bed, or better yet, in the morning or before your afternoon snack. Exercise in the morning, especially outside, helps set your circadian rhythm (Youngstedt et al. 2019).

Exercise for improved mental health

Stress, depression, and anxiety are very common issues. Some people are more affected than others. Sometimes the last thing you want to think about is exercising. For those who force themselves to exercise, they understand the rewards that come afterward. You've heard of the *runners' high*—that euphoric feeling runners have after a run. The same can be said for those who bike, try yoga, or do resistance exercises. Exercise can raise your serotonin levels (Young 2007). Serotonin is a chemical in your brain that can improve your sense of happiness.

When you're feeling stressed, depressed, or anxious go for a walk. Exercise is the best medicine. It will boost your mood.

I understand how hard it can be to try something new or to pick yourself up off the couch when you're feeling blue. Try it. Please.

Exercise for your immune system health

Exercise has a profound impact on your immune system. For example, mild to moderate exercise can boost your *natural killer T-cell* levels. These are the cells that help fight against viruses. Exercise also augments your *immuno-surveillance* by helping your white blood cells become better at seeking out and destroying viral invaders.

Exercise reduces chronic inflammation (elevated interleukins, cytokines, etc) to keep your immune system functioning, but not hyper-functional, to improve your health. It also has potent systemic anti-inflammatory effects because it affects multiple pathways and systems in your body (Nieman and Wentz 2019).

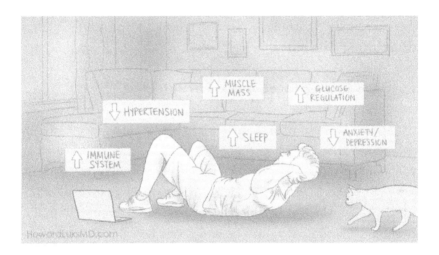

Exercise for your blood pressure

People with high blood pressure (hypertension) are at higher risk of several conditions, including heart disease, stroke, and kidney disease. One of the reasons is because of a type of receptor we call ACE2. The ACE2 receptors and an intricate blood pressure control system we refer to as RAS are important in moderating our blood pressure (Nunes-Silva et al. 2017). This may seem deep in the weeds, but it's relevant because of the role exercise plays in how ACE2 and RAS work.

By influencing RAS, exercise leads to widening (dilation) of your blood vessels, which decreases your blood pressure. The effect is so significant that your blood pressure can stay lower for up to 24 hours. Although the science behind why your risk diminishes with better blood pressure control is very complex, it is clear that the lower your blood pressure is (within a normal range), the lower your risk of many chronic disease states, thus improving your healthspan.

Exercise for heart health

Exercise also improves the function of your heart. Your heart is a muscle. If you exercise a muscle it becomes stronger and more efficient. The more efficient your heart is, the less it needs to work and the more reserve capacity you have. Many folks operate at maximal capacity just to complete their daily tasks. For example they may get short of breath walking stairs. Your *reserve capacity* is your ability to push harder, work harder, and walk more without feeling exhausted, short of breath, and in need of a rest period. The more excess capacity you have, the better your chances at combating disease.

A crucial tip when starting an exercise routine is to go slow. Don't push too hard or overdo it. Start light and work your way up.

Exercise is one of the best preventative strategies we have. Be proactive. Get up and do something that gets your legs and arms moving, and gets your heart rate up a bit.

Make your exercise a family event. Have a neighbor who will join you? Great!

Preparation for a longer healthspan starts in your thirties and keeps going for decades to come. Start being active as soon as possible.

Three pillars of an exercise program

Below are the three pillars of a complete exercise program. When considering what types of exercise to perform, it is useful to know what forms of exercise are available and the benefits that each provides:

- Aerobic (AET).
- Resistance, e.g., weights or bodyweight exercises (RET).
- Balance training or mobility exercises.

Types of exercise and their intended benefits

Aerobic exercise (AET) can be brisk walking, swimming, cycling, elliptical, rowing machine, running, or hiking. Some of the benefits of aerobic exercise are that it is critical to decreasing psychological stress, lowering your blood pressure, improving your insulin resistance, and decreasing your risk of cardiac disease, stroke, and type 2 diabetes. This form of exercise does not strengthen muscles nearly as much as resistance exercise. We will talk about how to get started and build your aerobic exercise in chapter 8.

Resistance exercise (RET) involves lifting weights, yoga, and bodyweight exercises such as squats. Resistance exercise helps you build and maintain muscle mass. This is absolutely critical when it comes to healthy aging and decreasing your risk of frailty.

Sarcopenia (age-related muscle loss) will decrease your muscle mass over time. Although sarcopenia begins in our forties, the decrease in muscle mass can be dramatic by the time you are sixty or seventy. That puts you at risk for falling, increases your risk of injury following a fall, and delays your recovery after a fall. Poor muscle mass and strength will worsen after a fall, starting a vicious cycle downward. Resistance exercises are covered in more detail in chapter 9.

Resistance exercises do not require a gym. You can perform bodyweight exercise on your stairs, by getting up and down from a chair, performing a calf raise, etc. Many people find squatting to be very challenging, but I have seen eighty-year-old patients squat. You can do this at any age.

Balance training or mobility exercises are a set of movements that work to improve your balance and your agility, but also work to strengthen many parts of your body. (Have you noticed that you trip and stumble more often?)

You're never too old to do this, assuming your doctors say it is OK to exercise.

Starting to perform balance exercises in our late thirties and early forties is highly recommended. Our ability to balance starts to diminish in our forties, and falls are a very common cause of injury as we age. Have you noticed that you trip and stumble more often? You catch your foot on the carpet or stumble. Or you may not even notice these subtle changes. It is critical to incorporate a balance exercise program as part of an overall healthy aging strategy.

An emerging body of scientific research is starting to reveal that exercise should be used as a primary treatment to mitigate or lower the risk of developing many chronic diseases (Mcleod et al. 2019). A proper exercise program, which will be one of the most important things you do to decrease your risk of chronic diseases, consists of aerobic exercise, resistance exercise, and balance exercises. Exercise will improve your odds of recovering from an illness or surgery. In your later years, an exercise program started now may just save your life. Exercise helps us optimize for longevity and an improved healthspan.

Resistance exercise has been shown to influence muscle loss, type 2 diabetes, heart disease, fall risk, and cancer.

Of course, it goes without saying, if you have heart issues or other serious medical conditions you should check with your doctor first. Also note that some balance exercises are challenging, so if your balance is poor, hold on to something secure, or have someone monitor or assist you.

The bottom line is to try something you think you'll enjoy... whatever gets you moving.

Take-home points:

1. Exercise has many benefits, it decreases your risk of chronic diseases and helps to improve your longevity and healthspan.
2. In addition to benefiting your physical health, such as heart health and metabolic health, exercise also often benefits mental health.
3. A complete exercise program should include aerobic exercise, (AET), resistance exercises (RET), and balance training or mobility exercises.
4. Different types of exercises can benefit you in different ways. For example, aerobic exercises can help reduce anxiety and lower blood pressure, while resistance exercises can increase your muscle mass and strength.
5. It's important to find a form of exercise that you enjoy, as this ensures you'll stay consistent with your exercise.

Chapter 8
HOW TO INCREASE YOUR FITNESS AND TRACK YOUR PROGRESS

While exercising for longevity and an improved healthspan requires movement, it does not necessarily require running. But for the many who are inclined to take their fitness to a new level, this chapter is for you.

Whatever your long-term fitness goal is, let's use an example to illustrate. Let's say your long-term goal is to run a 5k (3.1 mile) race 6 months from now. Your first (really) short-term goal is to go upstairs and put your exercise clothes on. Your next goal is to be able to run 1 miles in under 15 minutes. That doesn't seem so hard, right?

Let's do this...

Start with your target heart rate

We can measure how hard you are working out using the five heart zones. Your first few weeks of training you might be walking, with your heart rate only slightly elevated. Remember, it doesn't need to be sweaty and painful. You don't want to push your heart too fast, too soon.

HEART RATE ZONE 2 VS ZONE 4

ZONE 5: MAXIMUM

ZONE 4: HARD
- BODY USES GLUCOSE FOR ENERGY
- OXYGEN SUPPLY DOESN'T KEEP UP WITH BODY'S NEEDS
- LACTIC ACID GETS BUILT UP AS A RESULT

ZONE 3: MODERATE

ZONE 2: LIGHT
- BODY IS BURNING FAT FOR ENERGY
- BODY HAS AVAILABLE ALL THE OXYGEN IT NEEDS

ZONE 1: VERY LIGHT

How do you know how hard you're working out, and which zone you are in while working out? The first thing to do is figure out your target heart rate. Here's a quick rough calculation. How old are you? Subtract your age from 221. That very roughly approximates your maximum heart rate, although there is a high margin for error. You never want to get close to your maximum heart rate. Now, what is 70 percent of your maximum heart rate? That's:

- Your target heart rate = (221 - your age) * 0.70

Using your heart rate is probably your best way to identify what zone you are in. When you are in Zone 2, your heart rate is somewhere between 60-75 percent of your maximum heart rate. For an accurate assessment, we need to know your maximum heart rate and your resting heart rate (AHA 2021). I've hit my max HR on some trail races—a most unpleasant experience! Your resting heart rate is your heart rate in bed as soon as you wake up and before you get up.

If you know your maximum heart rate and your resting heart rate, TrainingPeaks® and other companies and websites offer calculators. My Zone 2 calculates out to be 126-139. With respect to your perceived effort, near the top end of Zone 2, you may find it harder to hold a conversation without having to pause to breathe.

Base building

One way to improve your performance when working out is a process called base building. If you are trying to run but are short of breath, then you need to walk for the first few weeks until your heart and lung capacity are built up enough for you to be able to run and still be able to talk. Seventy percent of your maximum heart rate *or lower* is your target heart rate as we begin. Any higher and the effort will be too painful and too stressful. Don't have a heart monitor? No problem. If you are walking fast or running and you are able to carry on an easy conversation without having to catch your breath, then you are probably under the 70 percent threshold. That's where you want to be.

This is called *base building*. We are getting your heart and lungs ready to begin an exercise program. Base building involves improving your body's efficiency and ability to put down a certain distance, at a certain pace, all the while using less oxygen and less energy.

The basics of base building, also called base training, involve low heart rate training. It means that for the first few months of your training you are concentrating on improving the way your body stores and converts energy using aerobic metabolism. You will build more metabolic machinery within your cells to handle the energy request from the muscles and you will be able to manufacture more energy when it is needed. You can only accomplish this effectively by base training. Your mitochondria not only determine your metabolic health, they determine your fitness level. Walking and running will increase the number of mitochondria you have, improve the blood supply to your muscles, and increase the efficiency of your mitochondria. We are going to go into more detail about your mitochondria soon.

Some of the fastest runners of our time train at a very slow pace. Unfortunately, most beginner or intermediate runners run too fast, too often. This is why understanding the basics of base building is critical. Even seasoned runners make this error far too often. Their slow runs are too fast, and their fast runs aren't fast enough.

Base building actually takes months. Do not plan on increasing your mileage too much until your base is built. Remember, even elite professional runners go through a base-building process!

Many sports scientists agree that many overuse running injuries are merely a training error. If you try to train too fast too soon, you run the risk of sidelining yourself due to injuries. Give me a few minutes and hopefully, you will understand why slower is often better. Again, the elite marathon champions of our time complete the majority of their training at a relatively slow pace.

Whether you start by walking one mile three days a week or two miles four days a week, just make sure that the intensity is set to *easy mode* if you use a treadmill. Again, that means that you could carry on a conversation during the entire walk. If you become short of breath, slow down or stop and recover. When I first started running I fell into the trap of running too fast, too often. Worse, I achieved a high heart rate far too soon. I blew through zones 1,2 and 3 as soon as I started. When I took base building seriously I was very discouraged. In order to keep my heart rate under 128-130 I had to walk often, and walk every hill. Many years later I am now realizing all the benefits of having a solid base to build on. I can run many hills and even more challenging terrains while keeping my heart rate low.

Base training involves long slow runs where your heart rate stays in Zone 2 or very low Zone 3. More about these soon. These are *aerobic* zones, and you should theoretically be able to run forever in these zones as long as fat and glucose are available. The waste that your muscles cells generate during aerobic metabolism is CO_2, which your lungs can exhale. This is a very efficient process. Lactate builds with more intense efforts. So if you are short of breath, you are building up lactate which will tire you out.

Building up to your fitness goals

Once you have walked a few miles at a brisk pace and controlled your intensity, then you are ready to try to run the same distance—if your goal is to run. The same concept of an easy intensity applies. When you transition from walking to running you might find that you need to run-walk-run-walk, to keep your heart rate at 70 percent or below and be able to carry on a conversation. As the days go by you will find that you are running farther than you are walking! And within a month you have hit your goal of running two miles at an eleven minute per mile pace or better. Be content, be proud, and let's move on.

Even though your walks or runs do not exhaust you and are relatively easy to accomplish, you will still get a runner's high. You will feel great and you will be able to stick to your new program.

The next goal is to build your mileage no more than 10-15 percent per week. That seems to be the amount that your heart, lungs, bones, and tendons can handle. At this stage of the game we do not perform any more strenuous runs or walks until your base is built and your mileage is up to 3.1 miles or 5k.

See, that 5k goal isn't too far away! After that you can explore how to improve your time and how to add on more strenuous runs. But until this becomes something that you look forward to, and find enjoyable, you might set yourself up for failure if you turn up the volume too fast.

If you have a personal or family history of heart disease or sudden cardiac death, please check with your doctor before starting any strenuous exercise program.

Zone 2 heart rate training for performance and a longer healthspan

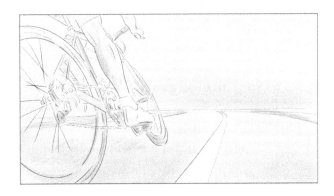

Many of us want to improve our athletic fitness, endurance, and performance. Face it, we also want to live longer, and with fewer health problems. That's where Zone 2 heart rate training comes into play. Not only will Zone 2 training boost your performance, it just might save your life. After all, your heart is just a muscle. In this section, we are going to dive deep into why Zone 2 HR training is a powerful tool to promote longevity and to keep you on the road for years to come.

"Train slow to run fast." The training regimens of some of our greatest athletes can teach us a lot. Zone 2 training involves training at a lower intensity (low heart rate) for a longer period of time. The science behind Zone 2 training illuminates why this is true and why it is also one of the best tools we have to achieve metabolic health and longevity. Low, Zone 2 heart rate cycling, swimming, rowing, and running are also key to improving performance and minimizing the risk of developing stress-related injuries.

All elite athletes spend months Zone 2 training, or base building. At least 75-80 percent of their active training is also in Zone 2. Let's not assume we know more than those who train these world-class athletes.

We'll get into how to determine when you are in Zone 2 later on. For now, we are going to explore the benefits of proper training and the downsides of ignoring Zone 2 training.

Heart rate training basics

When you are running your heart rate elevates. Running without a heart rate monitor, most of us will underestimate how fast our heart is beating. Some people run by intensity. That's fine, but you might believe you are in Zone 2, yet you are in a low Zone 4 state. I've been in zone 4 before and been able to have a conversation that felt pretty easy. Why is this so important?

When you are in Zone 2 your body is burning mostly fat for energy. It also has available all the oxygen it needs. Your body will eventually switch over to burning glucose, but in an aerobic manner because the amount of oxygen present is high enough. Your body's most efficient way to get energy is to burn fat because your body prefers that. This is the premise of *aerobic metabolism*. But fat can only be used up to a certain level of activity.

When you rev your body into Zone 4 you are now making energy from *anaerobic* pathways. Your body is forced to create even more energy because of your exertion (Zone 4). Your oxygen demands rise dramatically. As your pace increases, your oxygen supply doesn't keep up with your body's demand, so you breathe even harder. Your body will now use glucose for energy, but it will not have enough oxygen so you will enter into an anaerobic state. When you use glucose in an anaerobic state, you do not get as much energy from each glucose molecule, and you build up products like lactic acid in your muscles. This alters the cell's ability to carry on that activity for too long; your muscles will tire out, feel sore, swell, and your ability to run at this pace is limited.

The benefits of Zone 2 heart rate training (base building)

The benefits of Zone 2 heart rate training include:

- Increase in *metabolic flexibility*.
- Lower resting heart rate.
- Decrease in blood pressure.
- Lower risk of injury.
- Improvement in insulin resistance.
- Increase in the number of mitochondria.
- Increase in mitochondrial efficiency.
- Overall improvements in your metabolic health.

Zone 2 heart rate training enables you to use fat as an energy source for longer, and more efficiently. Thus you preserve your glycogen (carbohydrate) stores for longer. Glycogen gets broken down into glucose (sugar) which serves as your fuel source for higher intensity efforts. One end product of using glucose is the production of excess lactate. With poor mitochondrial function (which we're going to dive into in the next section), the clearance of the lactate is slow and the lactate builds rapidly. Accompanying lactate is a hydrogen ion. That hydrogen changes the pH of its local environment, in this case, skeletal muscle, and it is the hydrogen that produces weakness and exhaustion.

Now lactate isn't as bad as you think it is. In trained individuals, they can shuttle the lactate back into the cell and use it as fuel! The mitochondria will take the lactate in and use it as fuel.

Metabolic flexibility refers to the ability of your mitochondria to utilize fat and glucose as an energy source (substrate). At low heart rates, your main source of fuel should be fat, not glucose. Poorly functioning mitochondria, which is likely to be found in about 75 percent of people, will result in metabolic *in*flexibility, or the inability to utilize fat versus glucose.

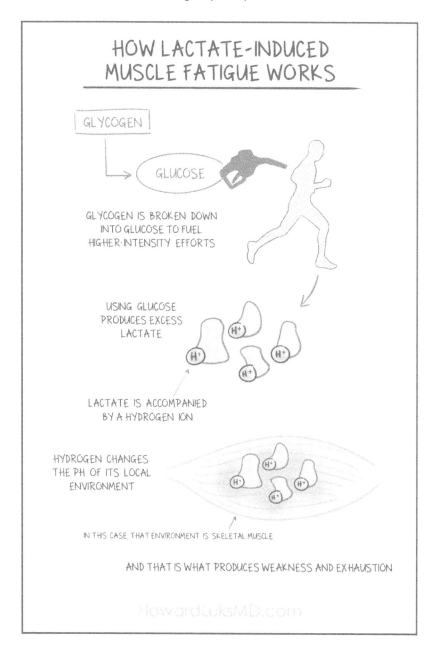

Perhaps even more important is that mitochondrial health is critical to longevity. As we discussed in chapter 2, many diseases that affect our lifespan are considered to be due to metabolic dysfunction, which, as we now know, is linked to mitochondrial dysfunction.

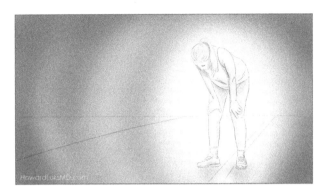

To understand why Zone 2 training and its impact on our metabolic health, we need to learn about mitochondria!

Mitochondria—the key to a healthier life

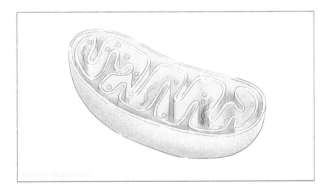

We are taught that the mitochondria are the powerhouses or "energy factories" inside our cells. Mitochondria are so much more, but we'll get to that later. We assume mitochondria are like an engine: give them fuel and they just work. Well, they are, sort of. However, like a fine race car engine, they require your attention to work in peak condition.

The healthier your mitochondria are, the healthier you will be. Poorly functioning mitochondria (mitochondrial dysfunction) is seen in people with metabolic syndrome, heart disease, dementia, type 2 diabetes, cancer, and so on (San-Millán and Brooks 2018). When it comes to your immune system, your mitochondria will dictate how well it will perform (Breda et al. 2019). Mitochondrial dysfunction is also one of the root causes of insulin resistance. Because nearly 50 percent of people have insulin resistance, this is a subject matter we need to pay attention to.

Poor mitochondria function is the root cause of chronic diseases, as we have discussed. Scientists are now finding evidence of mitochondrial dysfunction nearly 5-10 years before a formal diagnosis of type 2 diabetes is found in your blood tests. To elaborate, scientists are finding that a significant number of normal weight college students have signs of insulin resistance. Insulin resistance precedes a diagnosis of type 2 diabetes by 10-20 years. This will not show up on routine lab tests. It will show up on more sensitive tests. The bottom line is that the changes associated with poor metabolic health are staying under the radar for decades. But these changes are laying the groundwork for a substantial metabolic disease foundation for when these kids hit adulthood. This makes it all the more important to identify and deal with as soon as possible. *When it comes to mitochondria, the issues we care about are:

- The number of mitochondria you have.
- The metabolic flexibility of your mitochondria (in many diseases the mitochondria can only process glucose and not fat, so this inflexibility leads to significant downstream effects).
- Mitochondrial efficiency (how well your mitochondria process the various substrates–glucose, fat, and lactate).

Zone 2 heart rate training optimizes your muscles' mitochondrial function and minimizes risks of over-training

When you continue your base building (Zone 2) runs, your body will make more mitochondria in response to your training. Over time, you will find that your pace will improve, yet you will be able to stay within Zone 2 at these increased speeds. Initially, you will find that you need to walk up many hills or slow down often to keep yourself in Zone 2. This is essential work so stay with it. Forget about your pace, set your watch to show your heart rate zone or your heart rate, and adjust the intensity of your run according to your heart rate. Each week you will notice that your pace is slowly improving, yet you can stay in Zone 2.

When you have finished a base building program, your body will be far more efficient at creating and utilizing energy stores. Once you have completed the base building process, which can take many months, then you can start your special training runs such as tempo runs, progression runs, and fartleks (mixing periods of fast running with periods of slow running). These are all anaerobic runs. Running in an anaerobic state also has an essential role in the overall training of a runner, but ignoring base building and not starting off with the basics will leave you in a rut. You will be at a certain pace, and you will stay there. You should continue your base training by including a Zone 2 run in your weekly schedule on an ongoing basis. This will continue to improve your running efficiency, and it will minimize your risk of injury as you train.

To recap, when functioning well, our mitochondria use fat, glucose, and lactate as fuels. When your heart rate is in Zone 2 you are using fat as your primary source of fuel for energy production. But, how does this affect your muscles?

In our muscles, we have two types of fibers: Type 1 (slow-twitch) and Type 2 (fast-twitch). Type 1 fibers have plentiful mitochondria and prefer fat as their source of energy. Type 2 fibers are *glycolytic*, which means that they burn glucose. You'll recall that burning glucose produces lactate. Lactate can be used as fuel *if you are well trained*. But if you're not, lactate, and an accompanying hydrogen ion, build-up. It's the hydrogen that's the problem... lactate is actually fuel. The hydrogen ion will change the microenvironment around the muscle cell and make it far less powerful. You can lose more than 50 percent of your muscle power as hydrogen builds up. That is the hallmark of fatigue. Because we don't want lactate (and hydrogen) to build up and cause fatigue, this means that we want to use our Type 1 slow-twitch muscle fibers, as we do in Zone 2 training. Lactate will rise a bit, but it should rise to a point and stay there. The rate at which you fatigue will depend on how well trained you are, and how well your mitochondria clear the lactate.

Sometimes I rail against platforms that push us harder and harder each day. I want to stress: I am not against HIIT (high-intensity interval training). Let's call it a *concern* about how frequently you do it. By working out too hard and too often, over-training is a very real possibility, and a difficult problem to contend with once it's present. Along with overtraining comes an increased risk of injury. Recovery from injury takes a toll: emotionally, physically, and physiologically. A long recovery can affect us profoundly and should be avoided if possible.

How do you know when you are in Zone 2?

We are going to explore a very exciting way to identify your Zone 2 heart rate during your ride or run!

Let's say you purchased a bike or a Peloton® to optimize your lifestyle for longevity. Your new bike arrives. It looks sleek. You put your water bottles in the holders and jump on. You choose a class and pound out a 30-minute heart-thumping ride. You repeat this a few times a week. Certainly, this is good for your health, right?

Yes, there are benefits to high-intensity interval training, but... the importance of base building or Zone 2 heart rate training has fallen by the wayside for far too many of us. Our society loves quick, hard challenges. We gamify everything. You watch the leaderboard and want to move up further. Zone 2 heart rate training is hard, it's hard to run/ride slowly, but the payback is worth the effort.

Until recently athletes needed to go to a performance lab, or prick themselves to measure lactic acid to try and determine where they transitioned from aerobic (fat oxidation) to Zone 3 and above. That transition point goes by many names. We'll call it the *first lactic acid threshold* or LT1. Anything below your LT1 is considered aerobic. You are mainly using fat oxidation for energy production in this zone.

Heart rate variability

Your heart does not beat at a constant frequency; it varies. This is due to your autonomic nervous system. This is why heart rate variability (HRV) is a critically important marker of your physiological stress level. When properly analyzed in the context of training, heart rate variability can be key in helping athletes and sport enthusiasts monitor training load and further optimize performance. Even if you're not training, monitoring your heart rate variability with many inexpensive apps can be very informative.

Your heart rate is governed by many variables, including your nervous system. The nervous system has many working parts, and the *autonomic* nervous system is but one of them. Our cardiovascular system is mostly controlled through the autonomic activity of sympathetic and parasympathetic pathways. Analysis of HRV enables us to understand this control mechanism. Several studies on HRV highlighted how different features can provide insights into autonomic regulation and especially on *parasympathetic* activity, the branch of the nervous system mainly responsible for the body's resting functions (Sztajzel 2004; Thayer et al. 2010). Simply put, monitoring parasympathetic activity via heart rate variability can provide insights on physiological stress, with higher levels of stress resulting in lower variability. For example, in the context of sports, heavy training is responsible for shifting the cardiac autonomic balance toward a predominance of the sympathetic over the parasympathetic drive. This means that heavy training will typically reduce heart rate variability. Therefore, by monitoring it we can hopefully adjust and optimize training, reduce the risk of overtraining and ultimately improve performance.

How to measure your heart rate variability

Up to a few years ago, heart rate variability was used mainly by elite athletes and coaches or academic researchers working at the intersection of sports, fitness, health, and medicine. Today monitoring your heart rate variability is not just for athletes. In the recent past, many new, affordable, and user-friendly heart rate variability tools have been developed. These tools typically rely on commercially available phone applications with heart rate monitors (e.g., a Polar chest strap) to analyze data, compute the heart rate variability, and provide guidance to the user. You will see a drop in your daily heart rate variability reading if you are getting sick, if you are not sleeping well, or if a heart problem is acting up.

Given the technology available today, heart rate variability can be computed accurately without the need for any external sensor or device.

Prior to the appearance of the *HRV Logger* app, we did not have a well-proven means of determining when we were in Zone 2. We could go by how we felt... but that is often wrong. The HRV Logger app, as I will discuss, monitors your heart rate variability during your exercise. Every two minutes it gives you a reading.

The reading is your *DFA-Alpha-1* or *a1* for short. If your a1 is above 0.75 you are in Zone 1 or 2. If you are close to 0.75 you are nearing your *first lactic acid threshold* or *LT1*. Once you go below 0.75 you have left Zone 2 and are entering Zone 3 and beyond. This app has been a game-changer for me and many other Zone 2 enthusiasts. As I mentioned earlier, there are many times when I've run and was convinced that I was in zone 2 based on how I felt. I was wrong. My heart rate at my a1=0.75 is 133. So now I know exactly when I am in Zone 2 or beyond it.

The science behind using the *DFA-Alpha1 HRV Logger* app is very complex... and way over my head (Gronwald et al. 2020). This technology is available to everyone with a heart strap (preferably Polar) and a phone.

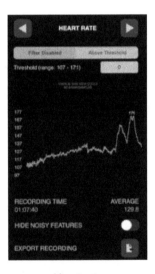

Heart rate

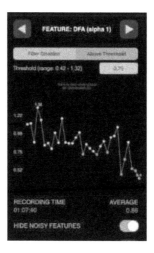

DFA Alpha1 for Zone 2 heart rate training

In the example above you can see a long Zone 2 ride with a heart rate between 105-137. The picture shows my DFA-Alpha1 as it was being displayed live on my phone. Your heart rate variability changes daily based on your sleep, as well as internal or external stressors. So your DFA-Alpha1 level of 0.75 will vary. One day it might be a heart rate of 135 and the next day it might be 141. Therein lies the value of this app. It enables you to stay in an aerobic zone and grab all the benefits and minimizes the chances of going into Zone 3 ("no man's land"). Many metabolic and other changes occur when you enter Zone 3, so if you are interested, try out this app and stay above 0.75 for your long aerobic runs and rides.

Cardiac drift

Cardiac drift occurs for most people near the end of a long run or ride. This happens when your heart rate starts trending up despite holding the same wattage on the bike or minutes per mile during a run. Dehydration can drive cardiac drift, but in non-elite athletes, cardiac drift is more likely due to metabolic stress. You are leaving Zone 2 and using more Type 2 muscle fibers. Those Type 2 fibers burn glucose and produce more lactate. The lactate causes your muscles to be less effective and consequently, you need to work harder to maintain the same effort.

What do you do if you see your heart rate drifting? As you drift, adjust your effort. Don't keep up the same effort. As your training improves, your metabolic flexibility, mitochondrial efficiency, as well as your muscles' ability to clear lactate will all improve. As your fitness level improves, you will notice that the time when you start to drift will also improve.

Breathing

If you can speak easily and in full sentences without having to pause at all you are probably in Zone 1. If you can speak or sing, but need to pause occasionally to breathe you are probably in Zone 2. If you cannot speak more than a few words before you need to pause, you are in Zone 3 and above.

This is a much less effective means of truly determining your exercise zones, but it is more useful than nothing. This is why the *HRV Logger* app has been so well received by runners and cyclists of all skill and fitness levels.

How long should I spend in Zone 2?

How much exercise is needed to improve Zone 2 fitness? Many professional coaches suggest that 90-minute sessions are needed to improve our fitness level as runners and cyclists. If performance is your goal, then preferably aim for twice a week. That's hard for many people to do, but that appears to be the right number. If you are pressed for time and want to get in a harder workout, that's fine. Try to ride 75-80 minutes in Zone 2 then crank it up for some sprints at the end of the ride. That way you are also exercising at your lactic acid threshold, and perhaps your VO_2 max in the same workout. In terms of cardiac health, short, high-intensity sessions are also important. It may be easier to perform these higher intensity sessions at the end of a long Zone 2 effort.

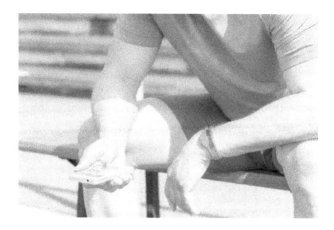

HRV4Training app

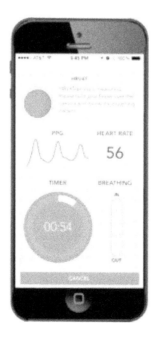

HRV4Training uses your phone's camera to extract photo-plethysmography (PPG, basically blood flow from the finger) and then determine markers of the autonomic nervous system activity, in particular parasympathetic activity. The technique has been clinically validated and proved to be a reliable measurement, as good as standard electrocardiograms with sticky gel electrodes (Russoniello et al. 2010; Lu et al. 2008; Altini 2015b).

By quantifying parasympathetic activity, the app is able to translate the information into an assessment of training load and provide actionable insights on physical condition, helping users to better understand how their body responds to training and other important factors in life (e.g., sleep, stress, etc.) (Garet et al. 2004; Pichot et al. 2000; Kiviniemi et al. 2007; Myllymäki et al. 2012)

From data to insights

Even with the right tools, heart rate variability can be difficult to gather under the right conditions, and especially interpret. Many factors influence heart rate variability, from body posture to respiration, age, genetics, gender, physical exercise, chronic health conditions, and more. So, how can we get reliable insights from heart rate variability data if it is affected by so many factors?

We do so in two ways. First, we need to look only at measurements with respect to ourselves, which means we need to collect a *baseline*, or a series of recordings so that the effect of different stressors is always evaluated with respect to what are our normal values, without looking much at the general population.

Secondly, we also need to control for as many of the previous factors as we can, and then evaluate the effect of what we care about. For example, in the context of optimizing performance, apps like *HRV4Training* provide a set of simple rules (or best practices) so that the measurements you take at home are as close as possible to supervised laboratory recordings, and your data is more reliable.

Best practices for HRV measurements

Here are a few best practices for short heart rate variability measurements that are very important to follow to get consistent results that can be interpreted correctly:

- Take the measurement of your heart rate first thing after waking up, while still in bed. This way you have a consistent time of the day and you are not affected by other stressors. (The only exception is if you need to empty the bladder. In that case, do it, then go back, rest one or two minutes to make sure your body is not affected by physical activity, and take the measurement.) Don't read your email before the measurement!
- Measurement duration: short measurements have been validated multiple times, and you can trust a sixty-second recording for rMSSD (time-domain feature) (Altini 2015c).
- Breathing is key. It doesn't really matter what breathing frequency you pick, but be consistent, use the same every time (Altini 2016).
- Body position: lying, sitting or standing are all good. What matters is that you always do the same, and if you decide to stand, be patient, wait a minute or two before recording since your body needs to be at rest.

Acute changes versus long-term trends

Heart rate variability is typically analyzed in two ways: acute heart rate variability changes and long-term trends (Altini 2015a). *Acute* changes refer to the easiest interpretation, for example, on a day following intense training, heart rate variability is expected to drop. HRV4Training will provide you with daily advice using a slightly more complex interpretation of this principle.

While it is definitely interesting to look at your heart rate variability on a day-to-day basis and understand the impact of intense training sessions, much research is now trying to use this data to understand more about our overall condition over longer periods of time, like weeks to months, in the context of a training program (Kiviniemi et al. 2007; Myllymäki et al. 2012; Plews et al. 2012).

Questions we can try to answer are: How are we adapting to a new training plan? Is our physiological condition optimal while approaching a race or should we change something? Are we at risk of overtraining or accumulating fatigue?

By combining a series of physiological parameters and methods we can definitely learn more about our physical condition. This is true regardless of whether we are a casual runner, a walker, or a trained athlete.

We can identify consistent patterns by looking together at:

- Changes in baseline heart rate variability (our weekly averages over time).
- The variability within our heart rate variability scores (for example if our readings are jumping around a lot during a week or are pretty much the same score every day).
- Our heart rate.
- Our current training program (training load and intensity).

Research shows that lower variability between readings together with a stable or increasing heart rate variability baseline can be more representative of good adaptation to our activity levels, while the same reduction in variability between readings when associated with higher heart rate and lower heart rate variability baseline is more representative of fatigue.

So in this context looking at multiple parameters can help better understand what is going on and tools like *HRV4Training* are constantly evolving to bring this analysis in the app and do the math for you, so that you can use the information to further optimize your exercise or activity levels.

Fitness trackers can change your life—If you let them

Can a fitness tracker nudge you into pursuing healthier activities? As we mentioned in chapter 4, sitting is the new smoking. People who sit down at a desk for hours on end appear to be putting themselves in a risk category similar to a colleague who leaves their workspace 4 times a day to light up.

Gentle nudges can be useful. Early on, trackers were fairly passive devices with very limited abilities to nudge us out of our chair. Now, my fēnix® 3 will not only track my runs and other outdoor adventures, but it will also gently buzz when it is time to simply get up and move. Even the Jawbone® and Fitbit® trackers have evolved to nudge us to move about. And with research clearly showing that these short simple strolls can add years to my life, I am willing to oblige. This concept of activity modification is the holy grail of the tracker industry. Certainly not everyone will care if their wrist is vibrating... but that's ok, I'll walk enough for both of us.

As a busy and observant orthopedic surgeon and sports medicine doctor, there is little doubt that I have noted a huge surge in tracker use. I have spoken to virtually everyone in my office with a tracker on their wrist and I have been very impressed by the fact that many admit that their tracker will cause them to modify their lifestyle to hit certain achievable goals. Of course, that's not true for all—but that's ok too, as no single technology is right for everyone.

There is no getting around the fact that we live in an always on and hyper-connected digital world. Many are enslaved by it. We document everything and take billions of pictures each and every day. Many of us will post our running or biking stats to Instagram®, Twitter®, or Facebook®. I've even heard some on the trails become very upset when their tracker malfunctioned and they were not able to post their run. It was almost as if the run didn't take place if it wasn't posted in the digital space for everyone to see. In addition to that, it is very clear that many of my virtual friends have been nudged to run after one of my posts, and vice versa. That is powerful.

Can a fitness tracker truly change your life?

The fitness tracker market is evolving at a very rapid pace. Gone are the days when your colorful companion counted your steps, and you then set the tracker aside until the following day. There are very few activities that are not trackable at this time. The research is becoming clear. The more we move, the longer we live. The more we know about our weight, body fat percent, heart rate, and blood pressure, the better we will be able to help our doctors help us. Any physician will tell you, we have seen many patients able to stop their blood pressure medications, diabetes medications, and more because they put a little effort into their health-related activities, so yes, if the tracker gets you moving, it can truly change your life.

NOTE: Do not stop taking your medications unless your doctor says to do so.

We can now track our:

- Steps
- Glucose
- Weight and body fat %.

- Blood pressure
- Mileage or effort from every sport imaginable.
- Heart rate
- Even our new baby's activity and breathing.
- Our posture
- Sleep

Actionable insights and fitness trackers

This is where trackers have the ability to change the lifestyle, healthspan, and potentially the life expectancy of those who need that little extra nudge. By receiving actionable guidance from your tracker of choice, you can make the decision to ignore or act— and I have witnessed hundreds of people take that little nudge and turn it into action.

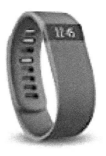

Fitbit®

This Fitbit® or an Apple® watch can track your heart rate and many other key metrics. Granted, many of you are shaking your head. That's all well and good. No single technology will be able to incentivize the population as a whole to get up and move. But those of us in the medical community will keep you informed of the technologies that are available if and when that light bulb moment occurs and you are ready to take active steps to living a healthier and hopefully a longer life.

Train wisely.

Recovery is a weapon.

Be better than you were yesterday.

Take-home points:

1. Base building, also known as Zone 2 training, involves increasing your "base" level of fitness, which is an excellent way to improve your fitness. This type of training involves training at a low intensity for long periods of time (meaning your heart rate is seventy percent of your maximum or lower) and can increase your healthspan and longevity.

2. When exercising, it's ideal to keep your heart rate at seventy percent of your maximum heart rate *or lower.* To calculate what your target heart rate is, use the following formula: Your target heart rate = (221 - your age) * 0.70.

3. Measuring your heart rate when exercising can be helpful, but you first need to know your baseline. That means you should measure your heart rate in a variety of circumstances, such as when you are laying down before getting out of bed in the morning, or when you're standing upright. Once you've established your baseline and know what "normal" looks like for you, you can then differentiate between acute changes and long-term trends.

4. Fitness trackers can be great tools in tracking your fitness levels. They can encourage you to move more and reach your fitness goals. Though fitness trackers aren't useful to everyone, many people have modified their habits as a result of using a tracker.

Chapter 9
MUSCLE STRENGTH FOR LONGEVITY

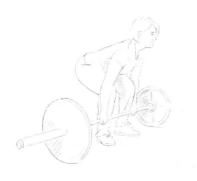

If you are over thirty-five years old, this chapter is for you and your future self. It is easier to prevent the onset of disease than it is to treat it. When optimizing your health and longevity, prioritizing muscle mass and muscle strength are critically important considerations. As we discussed in chapter 2, our muscle mass and strength naturally decline with age due to a process known as sarcopenia. The changes that occur to our muscles as we age can be profound. These changes can have dramatic effects on our health. Muscle mass starts to diminish as early as our forties. That's not old!

This muscle mass loss and the corresponding decrease in muscle strength ramp up dramatically as we enter our sixties. For example, grip strength is a marker of generalized weakness and can predict mortality. If we do not prioritize our muscle strength and muscle mass when we are in our thirties and forties, then the risks of muscle loss multiply and are harder to overcome—but not impossible—as we age.

Age is the number one risk factor for chronic diseases related to metabolic syndrome, such as insulin resistance, diabetes, dementia, atherosclerosis, stroke, and so on. Aging is inevitable. Evidence provided over the years shows that we can delay the onset of chronic disease by 10-20 years with lifestyle changes such as sleep, diet, and exercise. Over the course of this chapter, we will explore many of the benefits of a resistance and balance exercise program. But first, an important take-home message.

Frailty, falls, and hospitalization

Many people in their sixties and beyond suffer from chronic diseases. Diabetes, heart disease, and dementia exact a large toll on our lives. I see many patients who have metabolic syndrome (discussed in chapter 2), a collection of findings indicative of poor health. These diseases start to impair our health. This heralds the onset of a number of issues that have a metabolic etiology or cause. Weakness, muscle mass loss, and balance issues start far younger than you think. Chronic disease can lead to weakness and frailty.

Hospitalizations can worsen frailty in a matter of days to weeks. Unfortunately for many, the final common pathway to demise is often a fall. No, it's not the fall that kills you, it's the after-effects of the fall that lead to our demise. Stay with me for a second.

Chronic disease, over time, will initiate the onset of dementia and frailty. A fall may put you in a hospital for a few days. When you leave the hospital you notice that you are even weaker. Typically no formal interventions such as physical therapy or resistance exercise programs are initiated. You move less, the weakness worsens, the frailty worsens. You have trouble walking over a certain distance, and you have trouble getting out of a chair. The spiral down has started.

The next fall might cause a broken hip. The hip surgery and convalescence will exact an even larger toll on your body. At this point, you might require a nursing home because you can no longer walk unassisted. Your fall risk is now sky high, and because you are not moving around, you are prone to develop infections, pneumonia, worsening cardiac status, and worsening insulin resistance. You see where this is going. The fall that occurred months ago won't be the cause of death, but it will be the underlying reason for everything that followed in an eerily predictable manner.

Larger muscle mass is not only a friend to your metabolic machinery, it is a protective mechanism for your skeleton. As we age we also lose our balance more frequently. In our forties and fifties, we may simply note (or not) that we catch our feet on things more frequently or feel less stable when we stand or move abruptly. That is also a consequence of the aging process. It is this loss of balance and control that will ultimately lead to falls as we age further. Having greater strength and muscle mass will not only limit our fall risk but will also decrease the risk of injury associated with a fall. This is not a meaningless issue. While chronic disease makes us ill and frail, it is the injuries sustained after a fall which ultimately leads to further frailty and untimely demise. Each fall requires recovery. With poor strength and low muscle mass, each recovery never fully returns us back to our previous baseline. Each fall results in a little more loss of function. This sets us up for yet another fall, and a vicious cycle ensues.

Let's change this scenario. Now is the time to start a program to prevent it so we can break this cycle. Initiating and maintaining a good exercise program can help delay the onset of diseases. It is especially effective when combined with an emphasis on proper sleep and nutrition. Why is resistance exercise so important? To prevent frailty, weakness, and the risk of suffering from chronic disease at a young age. It is never too late or too early to start a resistance or balance exercise program.

Muscle mass is associated with longevity

Muscle and fat are two highly metabolic tissues. How our tissues interact with our metabolic machinery matters. Belly or *visceral* fat is very toxic to us, and we should seek to minimize the amount that we have. Visceral fat is responsible for considerable chronic disease states such as type 2 diabetes, heart disease, and non-alcoholic fatty liver disease (NAFLD). Muscles, on the other hand, improve our ability to manage glucose and have a role in mediating the severity of insulin resistance. Exercise is prescribed to people with insulin resistance or type 2 diabetes to improve glucose control and their overall metabolic dysregulation.

Muscle mass is linked to a decrease in all-cause mortality (Srikanthan and Karlamangla 2014). Simply put, the more muscle mass you have, the lesser your risk of dying from a chronic disease than some of your peers. It turns out that just one hour of resistance exercise each week leads to a decrease in all-cause mortality risk (Liu et al. 2019). One hour! You can do that!

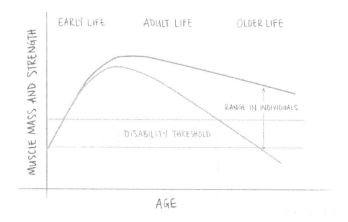

Muscle mass for improved longevity and health

How does our muscle mass affect our health?

As we know from chapter 2, muscle tissue is highly metabolic. That means that your muscles are metabolic machines that are always looking to burn fuel. By burning glucose (sugar) or fat, our muscles decrease the caloric burden our other tissues contend with. The larger and more active your muscles are, the fewer fatty acids and glucose molecules you have floating around inside of you. The fewer of these energy precursors floating around your blood, the less the chances are that those molecules will contribute to the belly (visceral) fat burden you have. Visceral fat can directly contribute to illness.

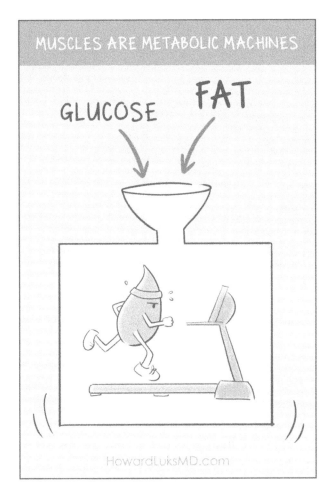

Visceral fat is the fat around your belly and is also the fat around the organs inside your body. Visceral fat, as opposed to *subcutaneous* fat which is the fat under your skin, does more than simply store excess energy. The metabolic activity of visceral fat produces far more of an inflammatory and toxic cadre of molecules that lead to chronic disease states. Visceral fat produces inflammatory markers. These substances increase your risk of chronic diseases associated with low-grade chronic inflammation. For example, we know from chapter 4 that heart disease requires both elevated LDL cholesterol and chronic inflammation to cause a block in your arteries. And as we discussed in chapter 3, chronic low-grade inflammation also increases your risk of developing dementia.

It should now be fairly clear why we want to optimize for an increase in our muscle mass over visceral fat. The larger our muscles are, the more overall metabolic activity is taking place. Muscles burn energy and do not "pollute" our bloodstream with toxic inflammatory chemicals. So the more muscle tissue you have, the more energy it will burn. That means you will burn more calories simply by having larger muscles. So to optimize our health and longevity we would prefer to have more metabolically active muscle than visceral fat.

Your muscle mass, or how large your muscles are, will directly correlate with longevity. Muscle mass protects your metabolism, enhances glucose uptake and energy expenditure. That decreases the number of excess calories that your body needs to store as fat. The less visceral fat you have, the lower your risk of developing worsening chronic disease. As mentioned in chapter 2, hyperinsulinemia is a leading cause of disease in our modern society. Hyperinsulinemia is a situation where your body requires more insulin to deal with a certain amount of glucose. This condition precedes the presence of type 2 diabetes by 5-20 years. Therefore, the more muscle mass you have and the more you exercise, the lower your risk of having hyperinsulinemia and progression to type 2 diabetes.

Face it, many of us fear dementia more than we fear heart disease. Neurocognitive decline or dementia is termed type 3 diabetes in some circles. That is because up to 30-40 percent of cases of dementia may be due to our lifestyle. Our metabolism and activity level affect many hormones that directly influence the health of our brain. Exercise induces changes in hormones which protect our brain tissue from degenerating (Tsai et al. 2015). Resistance exercise also decreases your risk of neurocognitive decline.

Improve strength to increase healthspan and longevity

Increasing your healthspan and longevity is not about having bigger legs for looking better. Nor does it matter what body type you have. Improving your strength is about improving your current quality of life and improving your chance of living a longer, disease-free life.

Improving your strength will decrease your risk of falling. You will lift your legs better as you propel yourself upstairs or walk downstairs. Your confidence will increase as your fear decreases. If you consider what your life will be like if you become frail, this sounds like a great reason to work out your legs if you're in your forties or fifties. As mentioned, frailty and falls are very common causes of demise. We should do everything we can to halt the progression of sarcopenia (the normal decline of skeletal muscle tissue with age). Your future self will thank you.

Resistance training reduces sarcopenia

As discussed previously, sarcopenia is one of the most important causes of functional decline, frailty, and loss of independence in older adults. When you lose your muscle mass you lose your ability to prevent a fall, and dramatically increase the recovery needed from a fall. Individuals who are already weak or frail are at risk of losing their independence if an unexpected illness or injury arises. Even a short 3-5 day period of bed rest might make it so that a frail person cannot recover.

Beyond falls and frailty, our muscle tissue accounts for more than 50 percent of our body mass and is essential from a metabolic perspective. Loss of this highly metabolically active tissue can have dramatic consequences for adults. Muscles help us control our glucose levels, use glucose as fuel, and have a role to reduce risks of insulin resistance and type 2 diabetes. Loss of muscle mass also contributes to poor health outcomes, fatigue, loss of function, disability, and death. Luckily, sarcopenia can be stopped in its tracks with an appropriate resistance exercise program and some nutritional support.

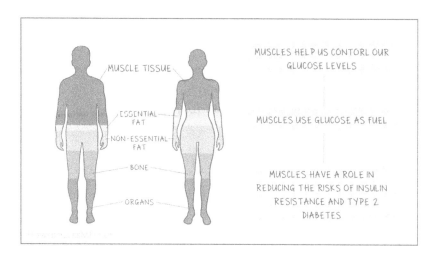

Everyone knows that exercise is important. Very few people, however, seem to understand all of the benefits that exercise provides. Many of the folks I meet in my office know the recommended exercise guidelines (30 minutes of aerobic exercise 5 days per week). They assume their heart will be the organ that will benefit the most. Most people do not understand the difference between aerobic exercise, resistance exercise, and balance exercise. Walking is a great activity, but it is not an example of resistance exercise. Many people will prefer a straightforward resistance exercise program over an aerobic program. In an ideal world, you perform aerobic, resistance, and balance exercises.

Aerobic and resistance exercise improves lipids and cardiovascular health

Many trials over the years have shown the benefits of exercise with regards to our heart (cardiovascular) health (Salehi et al. 2017). Aerobic and resistance exercise both have a dramatic effect on your cardiovascular risk by improving your lipid profile like lowering your LDLc and triglycerides while increasing your HDL. High triglycerides, LDLc, and low HDL are likely responsible for atherosclerosis and blockage of your arteries (chapter 2). By improving insulin resistance and glucose control you will have less chance of developing type 2 diabetes, dementia, and other chronic diseases. Those who perform resistance exercises will have less belly (visceral) fat. That will significantly decrease the chronic inflammatory mediators that are flowing through your bloodstream which will decrease your risk of hyperinsulinemia, fatty liver, and cardiovascular disease.

While muscle mass may not lower your lipid (cholesterol) level, you need to consider the big picture. In general, if you are conscientious enough to start a resistance exercise program to build muscle mass and to improve your health, then you are equally as likely to engage in other lifestyle changes to improve your health. This is how muscle mass likely associates with improvement in your overall metabolic health, the risk for chronic disease, and your lipid profile. For example, in chapter 2, we discussed how your triglyceride/HDL ratio can predict your risk of insulin resistance and type 2 diabetes. If you exercise to increase your muscle mass, you may increase your HDL (which is good). If you are now more conscious of your health and minimize simple carbohydrate (sugar) intake as mentioned in chapter 6, you will lower your triglycerides. That will decrease your triglycerides/HDL ratio and improve your overall metabolic profile. The same goes for diet and lifestyle in general.

As we've mentioned, the basic pillars of an exercise program include aerobic conditioning, resistance exercise, balance training, and for some, high-intensity exercise (HIIT). Yes, I mentioned balance training. Weakness and loss of balance increase our risk of falling. As mentioned, each fall becomes progressively harder to recover from. Minimizing your risk of falls, and injury following a fall, is directly related to muscle mass, strength, and balance.

While improved balance prevents falls, muscle mass and strength speed our recovery after a fall or injury. Sarcopenia that begins in our thirties is a brutal reality that requires active effort if we are going to try and break the cycle of decline in our function that starts to appear in our fifties. Starting an exercise program as soon as possible induces epigenetic changes that will affect lifespan (Rezapour et al. 2018). An *epigenetic modification* refers to the effects that exercise and muscle mass have on your DNA expression as mentioned in chapter 1. We have tens of thousands of genes in our DNA. Not all of them are turned on. Exercise leads to some of those genes being turned on (an epigenetic change), and those genes might decrease your risk of cardiovascular disease, insulin resistance, premature aging, neurocognitive decline, and so on. It is, therefore, never too early to initiate and stick with a resistance exercise program.

Muscle synthesis and muscle breakdown

Muscle mass and protein synthesis are in a constant state of flux. Our body is continually breaking down muscle protein (MPB) and rebuilding or synthesizing muscle protein (MPS). When breakdown exceeds synthesis, we start to lose muscle mass. This occurs on a micro-level (daily shifts) and a macro level (long-term shifts). Every night, our muscle protein breakdown exceeds our muscle protein synthesis. That's how rapidly this system changes. Achieving a situation where synthesis exceeds breakdown is essential to combat the changes that occur with aging and inactivity.

Building muscle mass is a very complex topic, but can be simplified for this book (Sharples et al. 2015). The three areas that we are going to focus on are:

1. Diet and appropriate protein intake.
2. Resistance exercise.

3. Dietary supplements to enhance muscle mass and muscle protein synthesis.

This is an all or none issue. In other words, we need all three.

We need to be sure that we are getting enough protein in our diet to stay in proper nitrogen balance, as mentioned in chapter 6. Your *nitrogen balance* is a fancy way of saying that you need to make sure that you have taken in enough protein, which is made from amino acids containing nitrogen. Protein ingestion gives you the building blocks that are necessary to synthesize muscle protein. Most adults do not get enough protein which limits their ability to build new muscle. You need at least 1.6 grams per kilogram per day (unless you have kidney issues).

Resistance exercise is critical, too, because building muscles requires a stimulus. You need to challenge your muscles if you expect to keep them. Muscles will respond to load or force regardless of your age. Yes, a twenty-year-old can build bigger and stronger muscles than an eighty-year-old. But an eighty-year-old will grow larger muscles if they perform resistance exercise too.

When it comes to supplements, you cannot assume that they work alone without proper nutrition and exercise. Creatine is a supplement suggested for most adults because it keeps our muscles larger and promotes bone health.

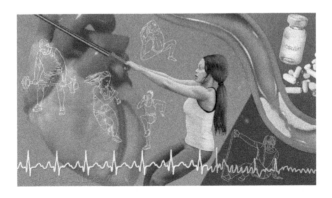

Resistance exercise has been proven to be as effective as aerobic exercise in delaying the onset of chronic disease such as dementia, heart disease, stroke, hypertension, insulin resistance, and type 2 diabetes.

As you can see, exercises that emphasize lower extremity strength and muscle mass can have a significant impact on your current quality of life and your risk of dying prematurely from chronic disease or injuries from a fall. As part of an overall longevity plan, resistance exercises have an equally important role as proper sleep (chapter 5) and a proper diet (chapter 6).

It is never too late, nor too early to start a resistance exercise program. You've got this.

I hope I have convinced you that maintaining or building muscle mass is essential. Let's dive deeper.

How to improve your muscle mass

There is no easy answer here. Preventing the age-related loss of muscle mass will require effort. We need to push and pull heavy things.

Recent research has shown that one bout of resistance exercise leads to muscle growth in ninety-year-olds (Fundazioa 2013). I often hear that folks are afraid of hurting their back, or something else from exercise. Well, we know that exercise does not worsen osteoarthritis. We know that most adults will experience back pain or shoulder pain, etc. throughout their lives. But the risk of not performing exercise outweighs the risks of injury while performing exercise under proper guidance.

To initiate a resistance exercise program, you need some guidance. Which muscles should you exercise? That depends on what you are prioritizing. For longevity and fall risk, you want to be exercising your legs, thighs, calf, and glutes. Those are our largest muscles and will have the most significant impact on our metabolism. Those are also the muscle groups that will minimize our risk of falling. If you think you are too old for these workouts, I have seen eighty-year-olds squat, and I have seen them push a sled across a floor at the gym.

For people in their thirties or forties, I know working out legs can be annoying. Try to embrace it. Squats, hip hinge exercises, and calf raises should be part of your routine. Runners, you must concentrate on calf exercises. Both seated and straight leg calf raises so you hit both of your calf muscles (gastrocnemius and soleus). Our calf muscles are one of the first to succumb to the changes brought by sarcopenia. It is essential to focus on them during our resistance exercise training.

Many people might benefit from a few lessons with a personal trainer to learn the proper technique. Others may benefit if they need that little push.

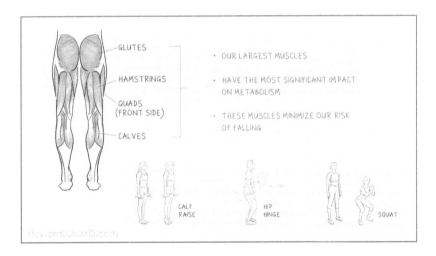

Start resistance training with your legs

It is time for us to prioritize activities and optimize our lifestyle to improve our quality of life and longevity. The more targeted and easier these discussions are to understand, the better the chance that you might adopt lifestyle modifications that could directly impact your chance of living a longer, healthier, more active life. No one wants to spend their last decade as a frail shell of the person they used to be. Your actions today will influence your risk of frailty in the future.

The muscles you choose to exercise should be those that will have the greatest protective effects. It's quite intuitive. You make your leg muscles larger. The larger the muscle the more metabolically active it will be. This will decrease your caloric burden and the amount of excess energy your other organs and visceral fat need to store. In addition, exercising your legs will improve your ability to prevent a fall, decrease the chance of injury from a fall, and improve your recovery time after a fall.

Larger muscles, or more muscle mass, improves our chances of living longer, happier lives, extending our healthspan and longevity. Larger muscle mass improves our metabolic machinery which decreases the burden of chronic diseases like obesity, insulin resistance, and type 2 diabetes. Muscle mass also correlates with improved recovery following injury or surgery.

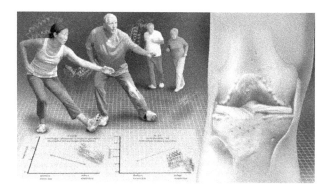

Why you don't need to be concerned about knee osteoarthritis

In case you're concerned about knee arthritis, don't be. Yes, knee osteoarthritis is a prevalent cause of pain, lost productivity, and disability. It hurts. And quite often, it hurts a lot.

Osteoarthritis of the knee has been increasing in terms of the percentage of adults who suffer from it. Thigh weakness has been found in people with knee osteoarthritis. Many scientists believe that thigh muscle strength *decreases* the risk of developing osteoarthritis of the knee (Øiestad et al. 2015). The precise reasons why exercise might reduce the risk of arthritic progression are still not well understood. Arthritis progression is a very complex topic. This is yet another reason why we should start to prioritize leg exercises.

There are many causes of osteoarthritis, and as of today, there are no medications or proven interventions that will prevent arthritis from getting worse. Therefore it is incumbent upon us to initiate appropriate changes to our lifestyle that will minimize our risk of developing osteoarthritis. A key take-home message is that walking and resistance exercise will not worsen the arthritic changes we see on your X-ray. Humans die of very predictable causes. Most of these diseases can be mitigated in terms of severity by exercise and remaining active. You are not going to protect your knees and hips by not exercising. That's not how osteoarthritis worsens.

Leg strength is also critical to aging well. So, simple leg exercises can reduce your risk of developing knee osteoarthritis, and possibly help you live a longer, healthier life.

Strengthening improves your stability, balance, and proprioception (the capacity to feel the position of a joint), all of which are known contributors to a decrease in injury rate. Injuries, especially injuries to the cartilage, increase your risk of developing osteoarthritis. Strengthening may decrease certain types of stress placed on the knee with our various activities.

However, the proper take-home messages are that thigh strength:

- Correlates with longevity and fewer chronic diseases.
- Improves how an arthritic knee feels (the stronger your

legs are the less of a chance that you may require a knee replacement).

- Is associated with a decreased risk of developing worsening arthritis after meniscus surgery of the knee.
- Has been shown to correlate with less painful knee arthritis.

Even though it hasn't been definitively proven to directly prevent knee arthritis from occurring, it is becoming more and more apparent that an improvement in thigh strength might decrease your risk of developing severe osteoarthritis in need of a knee replacement.

Are you concerned about starting an exercise program?

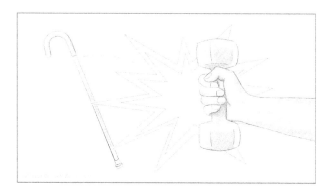

I often hear from patients in the office that they are afraid to exercise because they are so scared of hurting themselves. That is a reasonable fear. Injuries might happen if you perform resistance exercises. But you should fear the effects of sarcopenia more. You should fear the onset of frailty more. There is nothing worse than seeing someone inch along with a cane because they have lost their balance and strength. The risk of decline and demise from not exercising is far higher than your risk of injury.

And if you are concerned, of course you should discuss this with your doctor or cardiologist.

Can you handle resistance exercise? Probably. Should you check with your cardiologist first? Probably. Especially if you have a history of heart disease or shortness of breath.

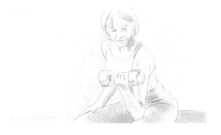

How much weight should I use and how many reps should I do?

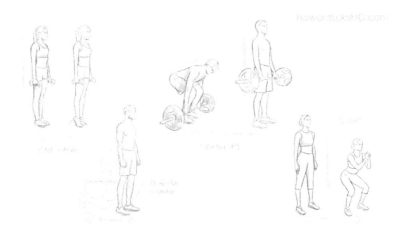

Leg exercise examples

There is a lot of confusion, even in the scientific world, with respect to why we should lift a certain number of repetitions. Consider this: Your *one-rep maximum* (1RM) is the highest amount of weight that you could lift with proper form only once. Many studies discuss lifting weights at 70 percent of your 1RM and doing approximately 5-7 reps.

Your muscle cells are actually firing, or active, to help you resist the load that you are working out with. If you are lifting a lighter weight you do not need all the different muscle fibers to fire or be active at one time. By increasing the repetitions until you are close to volitional failure you will be recruiting more muscle cells to become active as the muscle fibers which became active first start to become fatigued. The more muscle cells you have working, and the more muscle protein you will make, the larger your muscles will be.

The above argument is one of the reasons why we recommend weight lifting until you come close to the point that you can't lift any more (known as volitional failure). If you simply do 10 repetitions of a light weight that you find easy to lift, then you have not recruited many muscle cells or fibers to participate in your efforts. By lifting close to volitional failure you will recruit more muscle cells to contract or fire. That will lead to more gains in muscle mass. The key issue here is the concept that you do not need to lift heavy weights just a few times to failure. Instead, you can lift slightly lighter weights with more repetitions—as long as you go close to failure.

People like counting the number of repetitions they do. The reps that are easy shouldn't be counted. Instead, you should count the ones that are challenging. Challenge yourself. Do so wisely and with training to minimize your risk of injury.

Dr. Stuart Phillips has also reported that when recreationally-active participants performed leg extensions at either 30 or 90 percent of their one-repetition max (1RM) to volitional failure, there was an equal increase in new muscle protein synthesis (Burd et al. 2010). Therefore, it appears that reaching volitional failure is required for maximizing muscle protein synthesis and muscle growth. This can be achieved regardless of the amount of weight that you are lifting. Dr. Phillips concludes by saying that in contrast to current recommendations (ACSM 2009), he proposes that "an important variable to consider in regards to the optimization of muscle protein synthesis and the subsequent hypertrophic response is to ensure, regardless of the load lifted, that loads are lifted to the point of contractile failure."

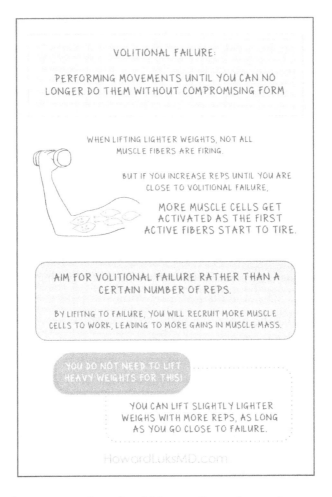

Resistance exercises should be performed two days per week. A balanced leg exercise program includes hip hinge exercises such as squats and deadlifts. Before doing them you should make sure that you know how to perform them properly to avoid injury. Calf raises are critical since the calf is one of the first muscles to succumb to sarcopenia. Bridges, leg extensions, and leg curls help to round out a balanced leg exercise program.

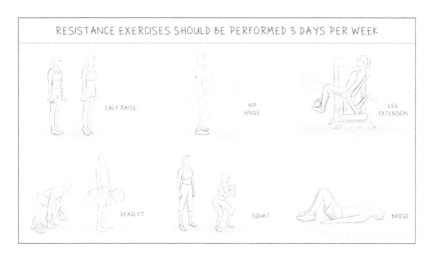

Leg exercises are even more important than upper extremity exercises. For runners, an exercise program can help minimize the risk of overuse injury. For athletes of all ages, resistance exercise helps with your power, strength, and helps decrease the risk of injury.

If you have any medical issues, especially heart issues, please check with your doctor before starting an exercise program. Be safe. Yes, injuries can occur by lifting weights, but the risks of injury are outweighed by the risks to your health of not exercising. Life is a series of risk-benefit analyses. Assess your risks and you will likely conclude that exercise should be a part of your normal weekly routine.

Diet and supplements for maintaining muscle mass

There are no magic bullets, and certainly no magical supplements, for maintaining muscle mass. There are some guidelines which help. First and foremost your muscles need amino acids from protein as we discussed in chapter 6. There are many recommendations online about how much protein you need to meet your daily requirements (Phillips 2015). Those requirements increase as we age. We need more protein to combat sarcopenia because as we age our muscle-building machinery is not as efficient. You may recall a reasonable guide for an average-sized person is to get 20-30 grams of protein per meal. That assumes you are eating three meals.

In addition to protein, if you are exercising, there is a fair amount of scientific research to support the use of creatine supplements to build muscle mass (Phillips 2015). Creatine works by getting into the muscle cell and bringing water with it which enlarges the size of each muscle cell. As you will recall, a larger muscle cell can generate more force, and a more massive muscle is physically capable of helping you avoid injuries following a fall.

Creatinine tells us how well your kidneys are working. If it rises, then your kidney's ability to filter out your blood is diminishing. Creatine will raise your blood creatinine levels, so tell your doctor if you are taking it, as this is a false elevation of creatinine. Creatine-based increases in blood creatinine levels do not mean your kidney function is diminishing. The creatine itself is metabolized into creatinine and thus can cause an elevation in your blood levels of creatinine.

Take-home points:

1. If you want to improve your overall health and longevity, it's essential to consider your muscle strength and mass.
2. Low muscle strength, low muscle mass, and weakness all increase the likelihood of falls; falling is a common cause of hospitalization among older adults. Unfortunately, frailty often increases at the hospitals, particularly if interventions such as physical therapy

are not initiated. Increased frailty often lessens one's longevity, if not lead to one's demise.

3. Improving your muscle mass can increase your longevity. Research shows that just one hour of resistance training a week can benefit you!

4. In addition to improving your strength and muscle mass, resistance exercise in combination with aerobic exercise improves lipids and cardiovascular health and reduces sarcopenia (the decline of skeletal muscles that naturally occurs as we age).

5. To improve your muscle mass, you need to consider the following: diet and appropriate protein intake, resistance exercise, and dietary supplements to enhance muscle mass and protein synthesis. In order to improve muscle mass, you need all three elements.

6. People of all ages should engage in resistance exercises. You can start resistance training using the weight of your body and doing exercises such as squats.

7. The cost to your health if you avoid exercise is higher than your risk of injury when exercising. You can start slow and exercise without putting yourself at major risk of being injured.

Afterword

As we've discussed, there is no one single quick fix to the answer to the longevity equation. There are definitely simpler ways to address health that don't involve rabbit holes such as coffee enemas, costly supplements, and quick weight loss schemes.

While there is no one recipe for success for everyone, everyone will find some piece of advice in this book that helps. You have to pay attention to what you're eating, how much you are sleeping and how much you are moving. Bottom line is that our bodies are meant to move, not sit still.

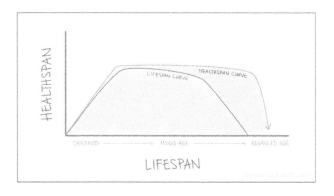

Remember that your metabolic health is an *area under the curve* issue. An *area under the curve* issue means that time is a crucial variable. The longer you are metabolically unhealthy, the worse your consequences. There is a Chinese proverb that says, "The best time to plant a tree was 20 years ago. The second best time is now." If you are in your 20s, 30s or 40s, the time is now to focus on your healthspan. If you are concerned... of course you should discuss this with your doctor or cardiologist.

In closing, my best "longevity simplified" advice to you is:

- Create a caloric deficit, then stay lean.
- Get sleep.
- Eat real food.
- Move often, throughout the day.
- Push and pull heavy things.
- Socialize.
- Have a sense of purpose.

About the Author

Dr. Howard J. Luks has been named one of the top Sports Medicine Physicians in the United States by US News and World Report and one of the Top Ten "Social Health Makers" for osteoarthritis. He has also been named one of the top Sports Medicine Physicians in New York for nearly 10 years in a row and one of Twitter's Top Ten Doctors. He served as an Advisory Board Member of the Mayo Clinic Center for Social Media for three years.

As a Board Certified Orthopedic Surgeon specializing in Sports Medicine, Dr. Luks' focus is on injuries that involve the shoulder, knee, and elbow. He graduated with honors from New York Medical College, completed his Orthopedic Surgery residency in New York in 1996, and a fellowship in Sports Medicine at the Hospital For Joint Diseases in New York City in 1997. As the Chief of Sports Medicine and Arthroscopy at New York Medical College and Advanced Physician Services, he is entrusted to teach the next generation of Orthopedic Surgeons about the needs of the child and college athletes, professional athletes, and weekend warriors alike.

More than twenty years of experience in an academic community has enabled Dr. Luks to offer a comprehensive sports medicine treatment experience including a good education about what's bothering you and a formal plan to move forward and back to your anticipated level of play.

Dr. Luks is a trail endurance runner and an amateur cyclist. You can find him on Strava and join him in his pursuit to always be a little better. He lives in New York and is a father to three wonderful children. They enjoy being outside as often as possible, which has led to a few fractures in the Luks' household.

Bibliography

Abboud, Joseph A., and Jae S. Kim. 2010. "The Effect of Hypercholesterolemia on Rotator Cuff Disease." *Clinical Orthopaedics & Related Research* 468 (6): 1493-1497. doi:10.1007/s11999-009-1151-9.

Achten, Juul, and Asker E. Jeukendrup. 2003. "Heart Rate Monitoring." *Sports Medicine* 33 (7): 517-538. doi:10.2165/00007256-200333070-00004.

ACSM (American College of Sports Medicine). 2009. "Progression Models In Resistance Training For Healthy Adults." *Medicine & Science in Sports & Exercise* 41 (3): 687-708. doi:10.1249/mss.0b013e3181915670.

AHA (American Heart Association). 2018. "American Heart Association Recommendations for Physical Activity in Adults and Kids." *American Heart Association.* https://www.heart.org/en/healthy-living/fitness/fitness-basics/aha-recs-for-physical-activity-in-adults

AHA (American Heart Association). 2021. "Target Heart Rates Chart." *American Heart Association*. https://www.-heart.org/en/healthy-living/fitness/fitness-basics/target-heart-rates#

Altini, Marco. 2015a. "Acute Changes in Heart Rate Variability." *Hrv4training*. https://www.hrv4training.com/blog/acute-changes-in-heart-rate-variability

Altini, Marco. 2015b. "Heart Rate Variability Using The Phone's Camera." *Hrv4training*. https://www.hrv4training.com/blog/heart-rate-variability-using-the-phones-camera

Altini, Marco. 2015c. "HVR Measurements: Duration." *Hrv4-training*. https://www.hrv4training.com/blog/hrv-measurements-duration

Altini, Marco. 2016. "To Pace, or not to Pace, That is the Question." *Hrv4training*. https://www.hrv4training.com/blog/to-pace-or-not-to-pace-that-is-the-question
Alzheimer's Universe. n.d. *Alzheimer's Universe*. https://www.alzu.org/

ACSM (American College of Sports Medicine). 2009. American College of Sports Medicine Position Stand. "Progression Models in Resistance Training for Healthy Adults." *Medicine & Science in Sports & Exercise* 41(3), 687–708. https://doi.org/10.1249/MSS.0b013e3181915670

Araújo, Joana, Jianwen Cai, and June Stevens. 2019. "Prevalence of Optimal Metabolic Health in American Adults: National Health and Nutrition Examination Survey 2009-2016." *Metabolic syndrome and related disorders* 17(1), 46–52. https://doi.org/10.1089/met.2018.0105

Arem, Hannah, Steven C. Moore, Alpa Patel, Patricia Hartge, Amy Berrington de Gonzalez, Kala Visvanathan, Peter T. Campbell, Michal Freedman, Elisabete Weiderpass, Hans Olov Adami, Martha S. Linet, I-Min Lee, and Charles E. Matthews. 2015. "Leisure Time Physical Activity and Mortality: a Detailed Pooled Analysis of the Dose-Response Relationship." *JAMA Internal Medicine* 175 (6): 959. doi:10.1001/jamainternmed.2015.0533.

Bell, Kirsten E., H. Fang, T. Snijders, D. J. Allison, M.A. Zulyniak, A. Chabowski, G. Parise, S. M. Phillips, & J. J. Heisz, J. J. 2019. "A Multi-Ingredient Nutritional Supplement in Combination With Resistance Exercise and High-Intensity Interval Training Improves Cognitive Function and Increases N-3 Index in Healthy Older Men: A Randomized Controlled Trial." *Frontiers in Aging Neuroscience* 11, 107. https://doi.org/10.3389/fnagi.2019.00107

Benetos, Athanase, Koji Okuda, Malika Lajemi, Masayuki Kimura, Frederique Thomas, Joan Skurnick, Carlos Labat, Kathryn Bean, and Abraham Aviv. 2001. "Telomere length as an indicator of biological aging: the gender effect and relation with pulse pressure and pulse wave velocity." *Hypertension* 37 (2): 381-385. doi:10.1161/01.hyp.37.2.381.

Breda, Cristiane Naffah de Souza, Gustavo Gastão Davanzo, Paulo José Basso, Niels Olsen Saraiva Câmara, and Pedro Manoel Mendes Moraes-Vieira. 2019. "Mitochondria As Central Hub of the Immune System." *Redox Biology* 26: 101255. doi:10.1016/j.redox.2019.101255.

Burd, Nicholas A., Daniel W. D. West, Aaron W. Staples, Philip J. Atherton, Jeff M. Baker, Daniel R. Moore, Andrew M. Holwerda, Gianni Parise, Michael J. Rennie, Steven K. Baker, and Stuart M. Phillips. 2010. "Low-Load High Volume Resistance Exercise Stimulates Muscle Protein Synthesis More Than High-Load Low

Volume Resistance Exercise in Young Men." *Plos ONE* 5 (8): e12033. doi:10.1371/journal.pone.0012033.

CDC (Centers for Diseases Control and Prevention). 1999. "Physiologic Response and Long-Term Adaptations to Exercise." *Centers for Disease Control and Prevention.* https://www.cdc.gov/nccdphp/sgr/pdf/chap3.pdf

CDC (Centers for Disease Control and Prevention). 2021. "Exercise or Physical Activity." *Centers for Disease Control and Prevention.* https://www.cdc.gov/nchs/fastats/exercise.htm

Collin, Lindsay J., Suzanne Judd, Monika Safford, Viola Vaccarino, and Jean A. Welsh. 2019. "Association of Sugary Beverage Consumption With Mortality Risk in US Adults." *JAMA Network Open* 2 (5): e193121. doi:10.1001/jamanetworkopen.2019.3121.

Courties, Alice, Jérémie Sellam, and Francis Berenbaum. 2017. "Metabolic Syndrome-Associated Osteoarthritis." *Current Opinion In Rheumatology* 29 (2): 214-222. doi:10.1097/bor.0000000000000373.

da Costa, Ianara Mendonça, Marco Aurelio de Moura Freire, José Rodolfo Lopes de Paiva Cavalcanti, Dayane Pessoa de Araújo, Bianca Norrara, Isleânia Maria Marques Moreira Rosa, Eduardo Pereira de Azevedo, Amália Cinthia Meneses do Rego, Irami Araújo Filho, and Fausto Pierdoná Guzen. 2019. "Supplementation with Curcuma Longa Reverses Neurotoxic and Behavioral Damage in Models of Alzheimer's Disease: A Systematic Review." *Current Neuropharmacology* 17 (5): 406-421. doi:10.2174/0929867325666180117112610.

de la Monte, Suzanne M., and Jack R. Wands. 2008. "Alzheimer's

Disease is Type 3 Diabetes—Evidence Reviewed." *Journal Of Diabetes Science and Technology* 2 (6): 1101-1113. doi:10.1177/193229680800200619.

Desideri, G., G. Castaldo, A. Lombardi, M. Mussap, A. Testa, R. Pontremoli, L. Punzi, and C. Borghi. 2014. "Is it Time to Revise the Normal Range of Serum Uric Acid Levels?" *European Review For Medical and Pharmacological Sciences* 18 (9). https://pubmed.ncbi.nlm.nih.gov/24867507/.
Diabetes.co.uk. 2019. "The Glucose Tolerance Test." *Diabetes*. https://www.diabetes.co.uk/oral-glucose-tolerance-test.html

Dolan, Eimear, Bruno Gualano, and Eric S. Rawson. 2019. "Beyond Muscle: The Effects Of Creatine Supplementation on Brain Creatine, Cognitive Processing, and Traumatic Brain Injury." *European Journal Of Sport Science* 19 (1): 1-14. doi:10.1080/17461391.2018.1500644.

Dunstan, David W., Robin M. Daly, Neville Owen, Damien Jolley, Maximilian de Courten, Jonathan Shaw, and Paul Zimmet. 2002. "High-Intensity Resistance Training Improves Glycemic Control in Older Patients with Type 2 Diabetes." *Diabetes Care* 25 (10): 1729-1736. doi:10.2337/diacare.25.10.1729.

Ebrahimi, Khadije, Alireza Majdi, Behrouz Baghaiee, Seyed Hojjat Hosseini, and Saeed Sadigh-Eteghad. 2017. "Physical Activity and Beta-Amyloid Pathology in Alzheimer's Disease: A Sound Mind in a Sound Body." *EXCLI Journal* 16: 959-972. https://www.ncbi.nlm.nih.gov/pmc/articles/PMC5579405/

Frontera, W. R., C. N. Meredith, K. P. O'Reilly, H. G. Knuttgen, and W. J. Evans. 1988. "Strength Conditioning in Older Men: Skeletal Muscle Hypertrophy and Improved Function." *Journal Of*

Applied Physiology 64 (3): 1038-1044.
doi:10.1152/jappl.1988.64.3.1038.

Fundazioa, Elhuyar. 2013. "Study on 90-Year-Olds Reveals the Benefits of Strength Training." *Science Daily. https://www. sciencedaily.com/releases/2013/09/130927092350.htm.*

Garet, Martin, Nicolas Tournaire, Frédéric Roche, Renaud Laurent, Jean René Lacour, Jean Claude Barthélémy, and Vincent Pichot. 2004. "Individual Interdependence Between Nocturnal ANS Activity and Performance In Swimmers." *Medicine & Science In Sports & Exercise* 2112-2118.
doi:10.1249/01.mss.0000147588.28955.48.

Gebel, Klaus, Ding Ding, Tien Chey, Emmanuel Stamatakis, Wendy J. Brown, and Adrian E. Bauman. 2015. "Effect of Moderate to Vigorous Physical Activity on All-Cause Mortality in Middle-Aged and Older Australians." *JAMA Internal Medicine* 175 (6): 970. doi:10.1001/jamainternmed.2015.0541.

Green, Kim. n.d. "Microglial Function in the Healthy Brain." *The University of California, Irvine.* https://faculty.sites.uci.edu/kimgreen/bio/microglia-in-the-healthy-brain/

Gronwald, Thomas, Bruce Rogers, and Olaf Hoos. 2020. "Fractal Correlation Properties of Heart Rate Variability: A New Biomarker For Intensity Distribution in Endurance Exercise and Training Prescription?" *Frontiers In Physiology* 11.
doi:10.3389/fphys.2020.550572.

Hagobian, Todd Alan, Megan Yamashiro, Jake Hinkel-Lipsker, Katherine Streder, Nero Evero, and Terry Hackney. 2013. "Effects of Acute Exercise on Appetite Hormones and Ad Libitum Energy Intake In Men and Women." *Applied Physiology,*

Nutrition, and Metabolism 38 (1): 66-72.
doi:10.1139/apnm-2012-0104

Hall, Kevin D., Juen Guo, Amber B. Courville, James Boring,
Robert Brychta, Kong Y. Chen, Valerie Darcey, Ciaran G. Forde,
Ahmed M. Gharib, Isabelle Gallagher, Rebecca Howard, Paule V.
Joseph, Lauren Milley, Ronald Ouwerkerk, Klaudia Raisinger,
Irene Rozga, Alex Schick, Michael Stagliano, Stephan Torres,
Mary Walter, Peter Walter, Shanna Yang, and Stephanie T.
Chung. 2021. "Effect of a Plant-based, Low-fat Diet versus an
Animal-based, Ketogenic diet on ad libitum Energy Intake."
Nature Medicine 27(2):344-353. doi: 10.1038/s41591-020-01209-1.
Epub 2021 Jan 21. PMID: 33479499.

Hooper, C., P. De Souto Barreto, M. Pahor, M. Weiner, and B.
Vellas. 2018. "The Relationship of Omega 3 Polyunsaturated
Fatty Acids in Red Blood Cell Membranes with Cognitive Function and Brain Structure: A Review Focussed on Alzheimer's
Disease." *The Journal Of Prevention Of Alzheimer's Disease* 1-7.
doi:10.14283/jpad.2017.19.

Ioan-Facsinay, Andreea, and Margreet Kloppenburg. 2018.
"Bioactive Lipids in Osteoarthritis: Risk or Benefit?" *Current
Opinion In Rheumatology* 30 (1): 108-113.
doi:10.1097/bor.0000000000000463.

Kiviniemi, Antti M., Arto J. Hautala, Hannu Kinnunen, and
Mikko P. Tulppo. 2007. "Endurance Training Guided Individually
by Daily Heart Rate Variability Measurements." *European Journal
of Applied Physiology* 101 (6): 743-751. doi:10.1007/s00421-
007-0552-2.

Konstantinidis, Klitos, and Erin Michos. 2015. "Exercise and
Cardiovascular Health." *U.S. News & World Report.* https://health.

usnews.com/health-news/patient-advice/articles/2015/08/10/
exercise-and-cardiovascular-health

Lai, Jianyu, and Joel J. Gagnier. 2018. "The Effect of Lipid Disorders on the Risk of Rotator Cuff Disease." *The Journal of Bone and Joint Surgery* 3 (3): e0018. doi:10.2106/jbjs.oa.18.00018.

Liu, Chia-Chen, Takahisa Kanekiyo, Huaxi Xu, and Guojun Bu. 2013. "Apolipoprotein E and Alzheimer Disease: Risk, Mechanisms and Therapy." *Nature Reviews Neurology* 9 (2): 106-118. doi:10.1038/nrneurol.2012.263.

Liu, Yanghui, Duck-chul Lee, Yehua Li, Weicheng Zhu, Riquan Zhang, Xuemei Sui, Carl J. Lavie, and Steven N. Blair. 2019. "Associations of Resistance Exercise with Cardiovascular Disease Morbidity and Mortality." *Medicine & Science In Sports & Exercise* 51 (3): 499-508. doi:10.1249/mss.0000000000001822.

Lu, Sheng, He Zhao, Kihwan Ju, Kunson Shin, Myoungho Lee, Kirk Shelley, and Ki H. Chon. 2008. "Can Photoplethysmography Variability Serve as an Alternative Approach to Obtain Heart Rate Variability Information?" *Journal of Clinical Monitoring and Computing* 22 (1): 23-29. doi:10.1007/s10877-007-9103-y.

Malhotra, A., T. Noakes, and S. Phinney. 2015. "It is Time to Bust The Myth of Physical Inactivity and Obesity: You Cannot Outrun a Bad Diet." *British Journal of Sports Medicine* 49 (15): 967-968. doi:10.1136/bjsports-2015-094911.

Mandsager, Kyle, Serge Harb, Paul Cremer, Dermot Phelan, Steven E. Nissen, and Wael Jaber. 2018. "Association of Cardiorespiratory Fitness with Long-Term Mortality Among Adults Undergoing Exercise Treadmill Testing." *JAMA Network Open* 1 (6): e183605. doi:10.1001/jamanetworkopen.2018.3605.

Martins, Catia, Linda M. Morgan, Stephen R. Bloom, and M. Denise Robertson. 2007. "Effects of Exercise on Gut Peptides, Energy Intake and Appetite." *Journal of Endocrinology* 193 (2): 251-258. doi:10.1677/joe-06-0030.

Mattes, Richard. 1990. "Hunger Ratings are Not a Valid Proxy Measure of Reported Food Intake In Humans." *Appetite* 15 (2): 103-113. doi:10.1016/0195-6663(90)90043-8.

McLaughlin, Tracey, Gerald Reaven, Fahim Abbasi, Cindy Lamendola, Mohammed Saad, David Waters, Joel Simon, and Ronald M. Krauss. 2005. "Is There a Simple Way to Identify Insulin-Resistant Individuals at Increased Risk of Cardiovascular Disease?" *The American Journal of Cardiology* 96 (3): 399-404. doi:10.1016/j.amjcard.2005.03.085.

Mcleod, Jonathan C., Tanner Stokes, and Stuart M. Phillips. 2019. "Resistance Exercise Training as a Primary Countermeasure to Age-Related Chronic Disease." *Frontiers In Physiology* 10. doi:10.3389/fphys.2019.00645.

Morton, Robert W., Chris McGlory, and Stuart M. Phillips. 2015. "Nutritional Interventions to Augment Resistance Training-Induced Skeletal Muscle Hypertrophy." *Frontiers in Physiology* 6. doi:10.3389/fphys.2015.00245.

Myllymäki, Tero, Heikki Rusko, Heidi Syväoja, Tanja Juuti, Marja-Liisa Kinnunen, and Heikki Kyröläinen. 2012. "Effects of Exercise Intensity and Duration on Nocturnal Heart Rate Variability and Sleep Quality." *European Journal of Applied Physiology* 112 (3): 801-809. doi:10.1007/s00421-011-2034-9.

Narayanan, Ramesh, Michael L. Mohler, Casey E. Bohl, Duane D. Miller, and James T. Dalton. 2008. "Selective Androgen

Receptor Modulators In Preclinical and Clinical Development."
Nuclear Receptor Signaling 6 (1): nrs.06010. doi:10.1621/nrs.06010.

Nedeltcheva, Arlet V., Jennifer M. Kilkus, Jacqueline Imperial, Kristen Kasza, Dale A. Schoeller, and Plamen D. Penev. 2009. "Sleep Curtailment is Accompanied by Increased Intake of Calories From Snacks." *The American Journal of Clinical Nutrition* 89 (1): 126-133. doi:10.3945/ajcn.2008.26574.

NIA (National Institute on Aging). 2017a. "Vascular Contributions to Cognitive Impairment and Dementia." *National Institute on Aging*. https://www.nia.nih.gov/health/vascular-contributions-cognitive-impairment-and-dementia.

NIA (National Institute on Aging). 2017b. "What Happens to the Brain in Alzheimer's Disease?" *National Institute on Aging*. https://www.nia.nih.gov/health/what-happens-brain-alzheimers-disease.

Nieman, David C., and Laurel M. Wentz. 2019. "The Compelling Link Between Physical Activity and the Body's Defense System." *Journal Of Sport and Health Science* 8 (3): 201-217. doi:10.1016/j.jshs.2018.09.009.

Nunes-Silva, Albena, Guilherme Carvalho Rocha, Daniel Massote Magalhaes, Lucas Neves Vaz, Marcelo Henrique Salviano de Faria, and Ana Cristina Simoes E. Silva. 2017. "Physical Exercise and ACE2-Angiotensin-(1-7)-Mas Receptor Axis of the Renin Angiotensin System." *Protein & Peptide Letters* 24 (9). doi:10.2174/0929866524666170728151401.

O'Connor, Anahad. 2015. "Coca-Cola Funds Scientists Who Shift Blame for Obesity Away From Bad Diets." *New York Times*. https://well.blogs.nytimes.com/2015/08/09/coca-cola-funds-scientists-who-shift-blame-for-obesity-away-from-bad-diets/

Øiestad, B. E., C. B. Juhl, I. Eitzen, and J. B. Thorlund. 2015. "Knee Extensor Muscle Weakness is a Risk Factor for Development of Knee Osteoarthritis. A Systematic Review and Meta-Analysis." *Osteoarthritis and Cartilage* 23 (2): 171-177. doi:10.1016/j.joca.2014.10.008.

Oikawa, Sara Y., Tania M. Holloway, and Stuart M. Phillips. 2019. "The Impact of Step Reduction on Muscle Health in Aging: Protein and Exercise as Countermeasures." *Frontiers in Nutrition* 6:75. doi: 10.3389/fnut.2019.00075. PMID: 31179284; PMCID: PMC6543894.

Paddon-Jones, Douglas, and Blake B. Rasmussen. 2009. "Dietary Protein Recommendations and the Prevention of Sarcopenia." *Current Opinion in Clinical Nutrition & Metabolic Care* 12 (1): 86-90. doi:10.1097/mco.0b013e32831cef8b.

Phillips, Stuart M. 2015. "Nutritional Supplements in Support of Resistance Exercise to Counter Age-Related Sarcopenia." *Advances in Nutrition* 6 (4): 452-460. doi:10.3945/an.115.008367.

Pichot, V., F. Roche, J. M. Gaspoz, F. Enjolras, A. Antoniadis, P. Minini, F. Costes T. Busso, J. R. Lacour, and J. C. Barthélémy. 2000. "Relation Between Heart Rate Variability and Training Load in Middle-Distance Runners." *Medicine & Science In Sports & Exercise* 32 (10): 1729-1736. doi:10.1097/00005768-200010000-00011.

Plews, Daniel J., Paul B. Laursen, Andrew E. Kilding, and Martin Buchheit. 2012. "Heart Rate Variability in Elite Triathletes, is Variation in Variability the Key to Effective Training? A Case Comparison." *European Journal of Applied Physiology* 112 (11): 3729-3741. doi:10.1007/s00421-012-2354-4.

Power, Geoffrey A., Brian H. Dalton, David G. Behm, Anthony A. Vandervoort, Timothy J. Doherty, Charles L. Rice. 2010. "Motor Unit Number Estimates in Masters Runners." *Medicine & Science In Sports & Exercise* 42 (9): 1644-1650. doi:10.1249/mss.0b013e3181d6f9e9.

Prather, Aric A., and Cindy W. Leung. 2016. "Association of Insufficient Sleep with Respiratory Infection Among Adults in the United States." *JAMA Internal Medicine* 176 (6): 850. doi:10.1001/jamainternmed.2016.0787.

Price, Brittani R., Donna M. Wilcock, and Erica M. Weekman. 2018. "Hyperhomocysteinemia as a Risk Factor for Vascular Contributions to Cognitive Impairment and Dementia." *Frontiers in Aging Neuroscience* 10. doi:10.3389/fnagi.2018.00350.

Rabøl, Rasmus, Kitt Falk Petersen, Sylvie Dufour, Clare Flannery, and Gerald I. Shulman. 2011. "Reversal of Muscle Insulin Resistance with Exercise Reduces Postprandial Hepatic de novo Lipogenesis in Insulin Resistant Individuals." *Proceedings of the National Academy of Sciences of the United States of America* 108(33), 13705–13709. https://doi.org/10.1073/pnas.1110105108

Ramanan, Vijay K., Scott A. Przybelski, Jonathan Graff-Radford, Anna M. Castillo, Val J. Lowe, Michelle M. Mielke, and Rosebud O. Roberts, Robert I. Reid, David S. Knopman, Clifford R. Jack, Jr., Ronald C. Petersen, and Prashanthi Vemuri. 2018. "Statins and Brain Health: Alzheimer's Disease and Cerebrovascular Disease Biomarkers in Older Adults." *Journal Of Alzheimer's Disease* 65 (4): 1345-1352. doi:10.3233/jad-180446.

Rasmussen, Line Jee Hartmann, Avshalom Caspi, Antony Ambler, Jonathan M. Broadbent, Harvey J. Cohen, Tracy d'Arbeloff, Maxwell Elliott, Robert J. Hancox, HonaLee Harrington,

Sean Hogan, Renate Houts, David Ireland, Annchen R. Knodt, Kim Meredith-Jones, Miriam C. Morey, Lynda Morrison, Richie Poulton, Sandhya Ramrakha, Leah Richmond-Rakerd, Maria L. Sison, Kate Sneddon, W. Murray Thomson, Ahmad R. Hariri, and Terrie E. Moffitt. 2019. "Association of Neurocognitive and Physical Function With Gait Speed in Midlife." *JAMA Network Open* 2 (10): e1913123. doi:10.1001/jamanetworkopen.2019.13123.

Rawson, Eric S., and Andrew C. Venezia. 2011. "Use of Creatine in the Elderly and Evidence for Effects on Cognitive Function in Young and Old." *Amino Acids* 40 (5): 1349-1362. doi:10.1007/s00726-011-0855-9.

Rezapour, Sadegh, Mustafa Shiravand, and Mahnaz Mardani. 2018. "Epigenetic Changes Due to Physical Activity." *Biotechnology and Applied Biochemistry* 65 (6): 761-767. doi:10.1002/bab.1689.

Rieu, Isabelle, Michèle Balage, Claire Sornet, Christophe Giraudet, Estelle Pujos, Jean Grizard, Laurent Mosoni, and Dominique Dardevet. 2006. "Leucine Supplementation Improves Muscle Protein Synthesis in Elderly Men Independently of Hyperaminoacidaemia." *The Journal of Physiology* 575 (1): 305-315. doi:10.1113/jphysiol.2006.110742.

Robinson, Jennifer G., Kevin Jon Williams, Samuel Gidding, Jan Borén, Ira Tabas, Edward A. Fisher, Chris Packard, Michael Pencina, Zahi A. Fayad, Venkatesh Mani, Kerry Anne Rye, Børge G. Nordestgaard, Anne Tybjærg-Hansen, Pamela S. Douglas, Stephen J. Nicholls, Neha Pagidipati, and Allan Sniderman. 2018. "Eradicating the Burden of Atherosclerotic Cardiovascular Disease by Lowering Apolipoprotein B Lipoproteins Earlier in Life." *Journal of The American Heart Association*. doi:

10.1161/JAHA.118.009778. PMID: 30371276; PMCID: PMC6474943.

Russoniello, C. V., V. Pougtachev, E. Zhirnov, and M. T. Mahar. 2010. "A Measurement of Electrocardiography and Photoplethes-mography in Obese Children." *Applied Psychophysiology and Biofeed-back* 35 (3): 257-259. doi:10.1007/s10484-010-9136-8.

Salehi, Zahra, Kobra Salehi, Mahin Moeini, Mehdi Kargarfard, and Masoumeh Sadeghi. 2017. "The Effect of Resistance Exer-cise on Lipid Profile of Coronary Artery Disease Patients: A Randomized Clinical Trial." *Iranian Journal of Nursing and Midwifery Research* 22 (2): 112. doi:10.4103/ijnmr.ijnmr_385_14.

San-Millán, Iñigo, and George A. Brooks. 2018. "Assessment of Metabolic Flexibility by Means of Measuring Blood Lactate, Fat, and Carbohydrate Oxidation Responses to Exercise in Profes-sional Endurance Athletes and Less-Fit Individuals." *Sports Medi-cine* 48 (2): 467-479. doi:10.1007/s40279-017-0751-x.

Schubert, Matthew M., Surendran Sabapathy, Michael Leveritt, and Ben Desbrow. 2014. "Acute Exercise and Hormones Related to Appetite Regulation: A Meta-Analysis." *Sports Medicine* 44 (3): 387-403. doi:10.1007/s40279-013-0120-3.

Seals, D. R., J. M. Hagberg, B. F. Hurley, A. A. Ehsani, and J. O. Holloszy. 1984. "Endurance Training in Older Men and Women. I. Cardiovascular Responses to Exercise." *Journal of Applied Physiology* 57 (4): 1024-1029. doi:10.1152/jappl.1984.57.4.1024.

Sharples, Adam P., David C. Hughes, Colleen S. Deane, Amarjit Saini, Colin Selman, and Claire E. Stewart. 2015. "Longevity and Skeletal Muscle Mass: The Role of IGF Signalling, the Sirtuins,

Dietary Restriction and Protein Intake." *Aging Cell* 14 (4): 511-523. doi:10.1111/acel.12342.

Siparsky, Patrick N., Donald T. Kirkendall, and William E. Garrett. 2014. "Muscle Changes in Aging." *Sports Health: A Multi-disciplinary Approach* 6 (1): 36-40. doi:10.1177/1941738113502296.

Small, Gary W., Prabha Siddarth, Zhaoping Li, Karen J. Miller, Linda Ercoli, Natacha D. Emerson, Jacqueline Martinez, Koon-Pong Wong, Jie Liu, David A. Merrill, Stephen T. Chen, Susanne M. Henning, Nagichettiar Satyamurthy, Sung-Cheng Huang, David Heber, and Jorge R. Barrio. 2018. "Memory and Brain Amyloid and Tau Effects of a Bioavailable Form of Curcumin in Non-Demented Adults: A Double-Blind, Placebo-Controlled 18-Month Trial." *The American Journal of Geriatric Psychiatry* 26 (3): 266-277. doi:10.1016/j.jagp.2017.10.010.

Srikanthan, Preethi, and Arun S. Karlamangla. 2014. "Muscle Mass Index as a Predictor of Longevity in Older Adults." *The American Journal of Medicine* 127 (6): 547-553. doi:10.1016/j.amjmed.2014.02.007.

Stensel, David. 2010. "Exercise, Appetite and Appetite-Regulating Hormones: Implications for Food Intake and Weight Control." *Annals of Nutrition and Metabolism* 57 (s2): 36-42. doi:10.1159/000322702.

Sumner, Anne E., Karl B. Finley, David J. Genovese, Michael H. Criqui, and Raymond C. Boston. 2005. "Fasting Triglyceride and the Triglyceride–HDL Cholesterol Ratio are Not Markers of Insulin Resistance in African Americans." *Archives of Internal Medicine* 165 (12): 1395. doi:10.1001/archinte.165.12.1395.

Suzuki, Wendy. 2016. "A Neuroscientist Says There's A Powerful

Benefit To Exercise That Is Rarely Discussed." *Quartz*. https://qz.
com/592569/a-neuroscientist-says-theres-a-powerful-benefit-to-
exercise-that-is-rarely-discussed/

Sztajzel, Juan. 2004. "Heart Rate Variability: A Noninvasive Elec-
trocardiographic Method to Measure the Autonomic Nervous
System." *Swiss Medical Weekly* 134 (35-36).
Thayer, Julian F., Shelby S. Yamamoto, and Jos F. Brosschot. 2010.
"The Relationship of Autonomic Imbalance, Heart Rate Vari-
ability and Cardiovascular Disease Risk Factors." *International
Journal of Cardiology* 141 (2): 122-131.
doi:10.1016/j.ijcard.2009.09.543.

Time. 2014. "Ending the War on Fat." *Time*. https://time.com/
2863227/ending-the-war-on-fat/.

Torres, Susan J., and Caryl A. Nowson. 2007. "Relationship
Between Stress, Eating Behavior, and Obesity." *Nutrition* 23 (11-
12): 887-894. doi:10.1016/j.nut.2007.08.008.

Tsai, Chia-Liang, Chun-Hao Wang, Chien-Yu Pan, and Fu-Chen
Chen. 2015. "The Effects of Long-Term Resistance Exercise on
the Relationship Between Neurocognitive Performance and GH,
IGF-1, and Homocysteine Levels in the Elderly." *Frontiers in Behavioral Neuroscience* 9. doi:10.3389/fnbeh.2015.00023.
van Vliet S., N. A. Burd, and L. J. van Loon. 2015. "The Skeletal
Muscle Anabolic Response to Plant- versus Animal-Based Protein
Consumption." *Journal of Nutrition* 145(9):1981-91. doi:
10.3945/jn.114.204305. Epub 2015 Jul 29. PMID: 26224750.

Weeks, John R. 2011 "Population: An Introduction To Concepts
and Issues." *Google Books*. https://books.google.ca/books?id=
NgRZf1A63GoC&pg=PA162&lpg=PA162&dq=squaring+off+
the+lifespan+curve&source=bl&ots=CgXl6wf70h&sig=

_nzwd1HgSpRiCqDTLWYXb30LRIo&hl=en&sa=X&
redir_esc=y#v=onepage&q=squaring%20off%20the%
20lifespan%20curve&f=false

Werle, Carolina O. C., Brian Wansink, and Collin R. Payne. 2015.
"Is it Fun or Exercise? The Framing of Physical Activity Biases
Subsequent Snacking." *Marketing Letters* 26 (4): 691-702.
doi:10.1007/s11002-014-9301-6.

Werner, Christian M., Anne Hecksteden, Arne Morsch, Joachim
Zundler, Melissa Wegmann, Jürgen Kratzsch, Joachim Thiery,
Mathias Hohl, Jörg Thomas Bittenbring, Frank Neumann,
Michael Böhm, Tim Meyer, and Ulrich Laufs. 2019. "Differential
Effects of Endurance, Interval, and Resistance Training on
Telomerase Activity and Telomere Length in a Randomized,
Controlled Study." *European Heart Journal* 40 (1): 34-46. https://
doi.org/10.1093/eurheartj/ehy585

Willbond S. M., M. A. Laviolette, K. Duval, and E. Doucet. 2010.
"Normal Weight Men and Women Overestimate Exercise Energy
Expenditure." *The Journal of Sports Medicine And Physical Fitness* 50
(4). https://pubmed.ncbi.nlm.nih.gov/21178922/.

Williams, Laura. 2021. "What is my Max Heart Rate and How
Can I Use it in Training?" *Runner's World*. https://www.
runnersworld.com/health-injuries/a20791648/max-heart-rate/

Wingo, Thomas S., David J. Cutler, Aliza P. Wingo, Ngoc-Anh Le,
Gil D. Rabinovici, Bruce L. Miller, James J. Lah, and Allan I.
Levey. 2019. "Association of Early-Onset Alzheimer Disease with
Elevated Low-Density Lipoprotein Cholesterol Levels and Rare
Genetic Coding Variants Of APOB." *JAMA Neurology* 76 (7): 809.
doi:10.1001/jamaneurol.2019.0648.

Wroblewski, Andrew P., Francesca Amati, Mark A. Smiley, Bret Goodpaster, and Vonda Wright. 2011. "Chronic Exercise Preserves Lean Muscle Mass in Masters Athletes." *The Physician and Sportsmedicine* 39 (3): 172-178. doi:10.3810/psm.2011.09.1933.

Yeh, Chiu-Ping, Hsien-Cheng Huang, Yaju Chang, Ming-De Chen, and Miaoju Hsu. 2018. "The Reliability and Validity of a Modified Squat Test to Predict Cardiopulmonary Fitness in Healthy Older Men." *BioMed Research International* 2018: 1-7. doi:10.1155/2018/4863454.

Young, Simon. 2007. "How to Increase Serotonin in the Human Brain Without Drugs." *Journal of Psychiatry & Neuroscience* 32 (6): 394.

Youngstedt, Shawn D., Jeffrey A. Elliott, and Daniel F. Kripke. 2019. "Human Circadian Phase–Response Curves for Exercise." *The Journal of Physiology* 597 (8): 2253-2268. doi:10.1113/jp276943.

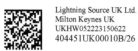